Cancer to Coma . . .
My Journey
Ciara O'Neill

This book is dedicated to:-

Mr John Rice

Peggy O Neill

Karen Davison

Acknowledgments

There are so many people to thank and to mention that it is difficult to know where to begin.

Firstly then I would like to thank my Family - Where would I be without them?

I certainly would not have been here to write this book if it wasn`t for the great care my mother gave me. My mother is a very special person. Having only just retired from her vocation of 40 or more years she devoted every minute of her time to looking after me and has been incredibly supportive.

My two brothers, Aidan and Shane, were also a great support. As were Katie and Liz, my two Sisters in Law. Finally, to my father, for being himself and my occasional McGyver.

To Karen Davison - A very big thank you to a very special friend who went above and beyond what could be expected of any close friend. Who looked after my dogs whenever it was required and for her extensive advice and help with this book, without which I would never have had the courage to undertake such an enterprise.

There are so many friends who have been so incredibly supportive to me during this time but I must single out both Niamh o'Donnell and Margaret Lane, who have been my friends now for almost 22 years.

Their support to both my self and my family has been invaluable.

To Bridie Murphy, my Home Help, who is a great person with a really good heart, who has taken excellent care of me and who has also become a very good friend.

Being blessed with a large wider family I must also send special thanks to Cecilia, Noel, Eileen and Nessa who have been in my corner since Day One of this journey.

A very warm thank you to Dr O Reilly for contributing to the book. For his medical care and being there when I needed him.

Professor Masterson for contributing to the book, for his magical surgical skills and for taking excellent care of me in Limerick Regional Hospital.

Professor Carney, for taking excellent care of me and his contribution to this book and Dr Grainne O`Kane for her contribution to the book.

Mr Rice for contributing to the book. For saving my life, taking excellent care of me and for all the support he has given me that will never be forgotten.

Mr Murray for taking really good care of me.

Denise Thornton for contributing to the book. For being a great support and a good friend, and my two District Nurses, Deirdre and Madeleine, who saw me through some very sore and painful days.

Acclaro Business Writing and Publishing for their editing skills and Elizabeth Mackey, for kindly donating her time and expertise in creating a great cover design.

To the Mater Private Hospital and the nurses in St Benedicts Ward – who were wonderfully supportive.

To all the staff of Kerry General Hospital who are far too numerous to mention by name, but to all of you, I am eternally grateful to each and everyone whom I have met.

Finally, Vistakon, who have proved to be the very model of caring employers. A big thank you also to Kate and all my friends and colleagues, as well as the management.

8

Table of Contents

Preface

I have a rare type of cancer called Osteosarcoma. It is a type of bone cancer which typically occurs in younger people, predominantly those of the male sex. But then I was never your average type of lady. Luckily, I have a close network of very good friends and a great family behind me, and this has been something that has managed to sustain me during the personal battle I have waged with this disease.

Before discovering the presence of this disease, my life had been pretty non-eventful. I had never been seriously sick before and I guess that it is only natural to take life for granted, until something happens to you which makes you aware of the fragility of it all.

So here I was, at 29 years of age. I had been suffering from a severe pain in my leg for almost two years, which had gradually worsened over time. The first time I went to see a doctor, the pain was attributed to a clot and I was sent to the nearby regional hospital for further analysis. This diagnosis was subsequently dismissed by them and no further action was taken to investigate the cause of the pain. As the pain continued to worsen, I went to visit another GP who diagnosed bursitis. The bursa is a buffer between the tendons and the muscles in the hip area, which can occasionally be prone to inflammation. So he prescribed me with some anti-inflammatories, saying that they should soon begin to work. Unfortunately this was not how circumstances turned out.

Around this time, the company I was working for was hosting a soccer event. I decided to take part, saying that I would stay in goal, as I could not run. Boy, did I regret that move! In the middle of the match I fell flat on my bum. Almost immediately, I knew that something serious had happened. The pain was so intense that it felt as if I had broken my leg. I lay there for a while. Eventually, I was able to get up and gradually put weight on my leg. I was really fed up and frustrated by this sense of having done a really stupid thing.

That weekend was a long weekend, and as I was not working and was able to put a little weight on my leg, I thought that I would just need a little bed-rest and wait for it to get better. However, a week or two passed and I was forced once more to visit the doctor, as I now found it very hard to sit, not to mind walk or run.

So I went to the doctor, and once again he

diagnosed bursitis, and prescribed anti-inflammatories. This time, however, he also wrote a letter authorising an X-ray to be carried out, although he did not appear to think that this would be necessary. He then referred me to a rheumatologist in the Bons Secours Hospital in Tralee. It niggled at me that I had lived with this pain for almost a year and a half, and it had still not cleared up. At this stage I heard from friends that the normal progression of events, when treating bursitis, is to get an MRI scan done, perhaps followed by surgery of some sort.

So when I went to the rheumatologist, she examined my leg and agreed with the GP, that it was indeed bursitis. I raised the possibility of getting an MRI scan done, but she felt that an injection of a long-acting inflammatory into my pelvic bone was what I really needed. Fortunately, that same niggling voice from before spoke a little louder this time and I asked for the tablets instead. I had to take them for three weeks. I told her it felt as if the pain was localised in the bone area, but again I got the feeling I was not being taken seriously. She felt that because I was able to put my full weight on my leg, it could hardly be bone-related, as if this was the case, I would not have been able to walk. It felt like I was back to square one again.

After a month, there was still no sign of the pain

abating. I eventually became so concerned that I decided to go to the A&E unit in Kerry General Hospital. When I got to see the doctor I told her everything and she was quite shocked that I had not already gotten an MRI to confirm the bursitis diagnosis. At this stage, an outpouring of frustration with the pain, and the length of time I had lived with it, resulted in tears.

So she wrote a letter to my GP saying that he needed to request an MRI scan to be done and also to refer me to an orthopaedic surgeon. She said that considering it was an old injury, nothing would come up on the X-ray, and that the MRI should shed some greater light on the mystery. Now I felt like I was getting somewhere. I decided to go back to my old GP, Dr. O'Reilly in Ballyduff, as I knew him and I regretted having changed doctors.

A week passed before I got a text from the surgery requesting that I make an appointment, as the results were through. So I made an appointment for that evening. When I got there my GP told me something had shown up in the MRI scan, something like a calcification around the hip joint. Mention was made of a tumour which really got me worried. He gave me the name of a Professor Masterson, who was based in Limerick, and told me to make an appointment with him straight away. When I got home

14

I was really anxious, and was about to pick up the phone to ring him, when his secretary rang me first, giving me an appointment to see him early the following week. She told me to make sure to bring the MRI scans down with me. The feeling that this was more serious began to grow stronger. So much for it being bursitis anyway.

A note from Dr O'Reilly
Osteosarcoma in General Practice

This is one of several primary cancers of the bone and presents relatively uncommonly in general practice. The commonest sites for this cancer are the lower femur (thigh bone) upper tibia (shin bone) and upper humerus (arm bone). It can also arise in the jaw and pelvis. The early diagnosis is important to improve chances of effective treatment, but as the long bones or pelvis tend to be affected, obvious clinical signs are difficult to pick up on routine clinical examination. The commonest symptom is pain which is a deep ache and is easily attributed to less sinister muscular/soft tissue disorders. Other later symptoms are swellings and joint disorders.

It is important not to ignore specific chronic aches or pains, and failure to improve with usual anti-inflammatory medications or physiotherapy should set off alarm bells. Further investigation is advisable. This is usually an x-ray or scan which can pick up the tumour and appropriate referral to a specialist centre can then be made by the general practitioner. The treatments for osteosarcoma are most likely a combination of chemotherapy and/or surgery and people more specialised in these areas can extol the virtues of each.

In summary, bring your concern to the G.P. as early as possible and make sure the G.P. acts upon it as soon as possible.

Diagnosis

Time seemed to stand still. I felt deep down now that this could be more serious than I had originally thought. I told no-one, apart from my friend Karen, as she has always been an oracle of good advice. What if it was cancer? What type? Had it spread? All kinds of questions were floating around in my head. Karen stopped me in my tracks and said it might be nothing at all, and calmed me down to a certain extent. I said I would wait and see but deep, deep down something continued to niggle. I carried on working, to keep my mind off it, and that helped to a certain degree.

The next day Karen joined me and we went to Croom to see Professor Masterson. The journey was short, but it felt like an age. Karen said that she would wait in the car while I went in. The wait was excruciating and it felt like hours upon hours before he called my name. He seemed like a nice man, yet I was too anxious to take anything more in. He took the scans from me and had a quick glance, then he checked the hip itself and then he sent me over to get an X-ray, while he had a closer look at the scans.

It took me a while to find the X-ray department and it was some time before I was called. After the X-ray, I had to go back to the waiting room, which had to be the worst place to be, when all you felt like doing was either hightailing it out of there or just wanting everything to hurry up so you could hear your results.

After a while, I was called back in. Professor Masterson had a very calm but serious and concerned expression, and I was not sure what to expect. We both sat down and he turned the computer screen towards me and asked me to take a look at the X-ray. He asked me if I noticed anything unusual. At first I looked and did not take anything in. But slowly it became painfully obvious that I was missing an ischium (the bone on the pelvis that you sit on) on my left side of the pelvis. My heart sunk to the floor and I could feel myself breaking out in a cold sweat. I looked at him with fear and disbelief. He confirmed that it was cancer and he believed that I had lived with it for around two years. So much for bursitis.

He told me that I had to get a biopsy, CT scan and a bone scan, to determine what type of cancer I was dealing with, and whether it had spread to other bones or vital organs. He also needed to see if it was the primary tumour, so that a treatment plan could be figured out. All that kept floating around in my head was that I was going to die. There was no way that I could have had this tumour for two years without it having spread somewhere else. He gave me a date for the following week to have a biopsy done, so on that note I headed back to the car in deep shock. He said to go home, have a bottle of wine and watch a DVD, to keep my mind off it as much as I could.

When I went out to Karen, I was in such shock when I told her, that I barely remember what I said. I do recall that we were both very quiet on the journey back home. We discussed what I was going to do and whether I should tell anyone. I did not want to tell anyone at all, but I decided to tell my brother Aidan and my sister-in-law Katie.

I found it hard telling them because I did not want this to be happening to me and I did not want them worrying about me, as they had three children. They took it well. Aidan had a positive outlook and they were both very supportive. Katie agreed to take me down to get the biopsy, as I was not going to say anything to anyone until something concrete had been confirmed. No point worrying everyone just yet. I was still suffering from both shock and anger. I could not believe that I had been misdiagnosed for so long. I had to clear my mind of all this and concentrate on what was important. I took a few days off work to get the biopsy done, and two days later, I also got the scans done.

We went down early to Croom and it was a really long day. I had to be sedated for the biopsy, so it took a while to be released from hospital that evening. I was wrecked and worried. A year ago, I had a friend who had a brain tumour, and I thought I understood parts of what she went through. But the truth is, you don't have a clue unless you are actually faced head on with it.

The next few days dragged interminably. I had my scans done in Limerick Regional Hospital. Then back again to the waiting game for the results. I had never felt so alone in my life and there was no-one in the world that could help with that feeling.

My brother Shane was home for a while from Paris, and I told him. A few days passed and then I got the dreaded phone call to come in for the results. The next day, Katie and I set off. When I got there I was put into a room on my own, and after a while Professor Masterson came in. Basically he informed me I had Osteosarcoma, which is a rare type of bone cancer, which was slow-growing. Thankfully, it had not spread anywhere else. I was to go to Dublin to meet an Oncologist, Professor Carney, as he is the main expert in this country for these types of cancer. It was looking like I was going to have to have chemotherapy, surgery and then more chemotherapy.

Professor Masterson said he had a lot of research to do himself, to determine whether a prosthesis could be made, as half my pelvis may have to be removed. That was to be discussed at a later date. My head was numb. It was official. I had cancer and I had a 50:50 chance of surviving. Life was a bitch really. When you have been told you have cancer, something is taken away from you, you feel robbed and nothing will ever feel right again. You certainly can never take life for granted, as a certain confidence in yourself goes and you feel that your body has let you down in a big way. There is no switching it off in your head. It is always there, niggling away in the back of your mind. When I left, I told Katie on the way home. It was now time to tell the rest of the family.

I was dreading this part, as I knew that some people had started to treat my friend differently when she was diagnosed. I was afraid that would happen to me as well. So when I got home, I broke the news to my mother. I could see her shock and felt the rawness of her tears. At that moment I had to leave. I decided to go to Karen to tell her the news. I just could not bear to be around someone that was upset, because I felt that I had to be the strong one. Somehow I had to hide how upset I felt. I told my father and obviously he was shocked.

I told my two very close friends, Niamh and

21

Margaret. They were the best support a friend could have. I then drove down to work and organised to meet my manager and a person from the Human Resources Department and I broke the news to them. That was also hard, as I was afraid they were going to tell me that my position was no longer tenable. They were, however, fantastic. They were incredibly supportive, telling me to take as much time as I needed. They relieved an immense pressure from me and it was a great feeling. My mind had been swimming with visions of people who had cancer being forced to leave their jobs. But thankfully, I did not have to worry about that and it was a great relief. Vistakon is a great company to work for.

A Note from Prof. Eric Masterson
BSc.M.Ch F.R.C.S.I.F.R.C.S (orth)Consultant Orthopaedic Surgeon

Osteosarcoma is a devastating disease. It predominantly affects children and young adults and cancer is a diagnosis that never crosses the minds of people at that age. The devastation of the disease comes from two main areas.

The first is that the treatment involves quite

significant chemotherapy with the hair loss and associated illness and loss of body image that this involves. It also involves ablative surgery for the tumour in question and this frequently involves mutilating procedures which also have very significant affects on body image.

The second area of devastation with Osteosarcoma is that a young, previously healthy people are forced to confront their own potential mortality in a way that they have never before needed to do. Being told that there is a 50% chance of being disease free in 5 years time following successful conclusion of treatment can be seen as devastating to some individuals whereas others see it as a challenge. This is very much personality dependent and also is influenced significantly by the support of family and friends.

Chemotherapy

The moment that I received my appointment for Dublin, I was sick with nerves. You really do feel like you are on your own. I talked to my friend Clare. It was somehow easier to talk to her really, as she had been through it herself. I knew I was lucky that it was slow-growing and that it hadn`t spread anywhere else in my body, but I could not help feeling cheated. I still had to keep up a brave face in front of my family and friends, and waited till night time, when I was on my own, to break down and cry and let it all out. I don`t really find it that easy to talk about my feelings to anyone or to let my emotions show either. I tried giving up cigarettes but to no avail.

My mother and father accompanied me to Dublin and it felt like the longest journey ever. I drove most of the way, in a futile effort to keep my mind off things. Our destination was the Mater Private Hospital, where I was to meet Professor Carney. I was afraid as hell of meeting him. What was he going to say to me? Funny really, as this was a doctor that was a caring professional, as well as a human being, and yet the scary taboo that is cancer made me afraid to see him because he was an oncologist. I did not know what to expect from him really. This was all new to me. I also really did not know how to handle it either, truth be told.

We eventually found the place and my mother came in with me to the consultation room. We discussed how rare the type of cancer was, occurring in only around nine people in Ireland each year. Typical, that I would have to be the one to suffer from a rare type of cancer. Anything to be awkward! We then discussed the chemotherapy treatment and the likely effects of that. To tell you the truth, I probably only took in half that conversation.

I was to have four cycles of chemotherapy, with two different types of drugs. The first cycle was going to be methotrexate and I would have a two-week break after that. Then the second cycle was going to be rubicin. Following this, I would have a three-week break before returning to methotrexate for cycle three, and cycle four was rubicin and -------. I would then have a month off chemotherapy, which would be followed by major surgery. I would need a month or so to recover from that, and then back for another four cycles of chemotherapy. He may place me on a different type of chemotherapy drug after the surgery, depending on how well the first four cycles worked.

The objective of the first four cycles was to try to reduce the size of the tumour, and to kill as much of the cancer cells as possible. So fingers crossed. He also gave me the option of saving eggs if I wanted to have a baby afterwards, as the chemotherapy could reduce the chances of conceiving a baby. My head struggled to take it all in. Considering I was currently single, added to the fact that having this disease meant that I was not now likely to attract a nice fellow for myself, I declined the option of saving any eggs. I was, however, told that I needed to get an injection and that I would need to commence a course of tablets called Liveal, in order to protect my ovaries. These tablets function by putting you through an early menopause, though the effects are not permanent.

So I was to start the treatment the following week. I was sick with nerves with what was to come. So when I got home, I organised with Dr. O'Reilly to get the injection done. I began to prepare for the week ahead. I had organised for Karen to look after the dogs while I was up in Dublin. After day 10, I would have to have a blood test in order to ensure that my immunity level was OK and, if affirmative, I would be able to have the dogs home for a while before going back up. Anyway, that was the so-called plan, but I was told any patient who undergoes chemotherapy, should learn to expect the unexpected.

27

My mother was going to come with me and we were going up by train. My friend Niamh bought me a diary and I brought that up in the train with me and I wrote in it for a while. I could not distract myself though, as the thoughts of what was to come weighed heavily on my mind. My Aunt Sheila planned to meet us outside the hospital as she said she would keep Mom company (and offer her some moral support).

We met up outside the hospital, and having arrived early, we went for some lunch. Food, however, was the remotest thing from my mind. I ate a small bit and then suddenly it was time to go and get admitted. When I got there, everyone seemed nice, and I got bombarded with a long list of questions. I then had to get a blood test, be weighed and have my height checked. By this time, Mom had to go and check into the hotel, and besides it was time to settle in for the night anyway. So far so good.

The next day I had to undergo a battery of tests, a heart and hearing test in particular, as one of the chemotherapy drugs can affect hearing. I was set up with a drip line, and as I have incredibly bad veins, it was not easy for them to find one. I then got a beautiful delivery of flowers from my brother Shane in Paris. They were beautiful, but unfortunately I was being moved that evening to the oncology ward, and the flowers could not come with me. So my mother

28

brought them down to the church.

The next day was D-day. I eventually got some sleep and I was awake by 6am, because Professor Carney did his rounds then and he informed me I was having the chemotherapy that morning. Oh the joys! So sometime in the late morning, two nurses came in, all gowned-up with purple gloves and a tray. I will never forget the smell of alcohol from the wipes. They double-checked all my details and then they hooked me up to the chemotherapy drug. It was to go in for an hour or two.

My mother was great and thankfully she was bolstered by my Aunt Sheila. They kept me company the whole time and helped me keep things off my mind as much as possible. Thus far, I felt fine, and when the drip finished, I felt the urge to go out for a cigarette. When I came back up I felt a bit tired, but nothing too serious. I tried to eat something and I decided I did not like hospital food at all. That evening I felt a certain degree of nausea, though aided by motilium and valoid, I eventually felt fine.

The next day, Sheila left, and it was now just Mom and me. My father was coming the next day to collect me, providing the blood results were good. I had a blood test that day and all was good, so I was staying positive and was glad to be nearing home-time. I was in a room by myself, which suited me, because I was not really in the mood for talking to other people, and I was scared of hearing other people's stories of their cancer experience. In spite of all that had happened, I was still one big scaredy cat. I kept getting phone calls, which I would not answer, because I was not in talking form. The only call I made was to Karen, to see how my babies were doing, because I was missing them greatly. Cancer really isolates you, though I began to later realise that it only isolates you if you let it do so. At this particular moment, I did let it isolate me. But I think I needed to do so in order to keep up a strong front for my family and friends.

The next morning eventually came and Professor Carney said I could go home, provided the blood results were clear. So there was a long wait until the results came in the afternoon. By this time, my father had arrived and my bloods came back clear, so yippee, I was going home after having my first cycle of chemotherapy.

The week or so that followed went okay - I was sick and tired but not that bad. I couldn`t eat a lot and my mouth was under siege by mouth ulcers. They were really annoying and painful, which made it quite hard to eat. I had more blood tests and the results were good, so I managed to have my dogs back for a couple of days. It was great to see them and be around them again. My Mom could not stop fussing and it was

30

starting to drive me mad, but I knew she meant well. I couldn't believe that it was already nearing the time to go back up to Dublin and start the process all over again, but at least it was the second cycle and that meant I only had two more cycles left after that.

We came up by train again to Dublin for the second round. I was admitted a lot faster this time, but asked the same amount of questions and a blood test was taken. I settled in for the night. I was once again awoken at 6am to see Professor Carney, and he said I was going to be getting a port channel inserted before I started chemotherapy. This port makes life very easy when you have bad veins.

So I was brought down late that morning and I got a local anaesthetic, and they inserted the port into one of my bigger veins on my chest. After that, I was left for an hour to recover, and once again two nurses came, in all gowned up and purple-gloved. They double-checked my details and then hooked me onto the chemotherapy drugs. This time it took less time than the previous one and boy, did this one mean business. I was really sick. I vomited profusely and when I got home it felt as if someone had hit my mouth with a hurley, as my gums were really sore and my wisdom teeth ached. My ears hurt and any loud noises really irritated me. I could barely eat because of my mouth. I was living on soup, jelly and ice cream -

anything that had a soft texture. I had mouth ulcers at the back of my throat which were really nasty. My hair got thinner. I did not lose it but it was really thin, so I just cut it short and wore a headband the whole time. I was more comfortable that way.

The second round of chemotherapy was very tough and it did take an awful lot out of me. I don't think that I will ever forget the fatigue, nausea and sores in my mouth. I will never forget that week. I began to wish my life away at this stage, anything for a bit of a break from it. Eventually the symptoms subsided and I had my bloods tested and they were OK. I was happy to see the dogs once more. My ears still irritated me though; it took a while for that to settle down.

Well, I was heading into my third round of chemotherapy, and since I was resuming the methotrexate, I was hoping I would have it easier then the last one. Fingers crossed anyway. My Aunt Cecilia decided to come with us to keep us company, and it was nice having her on the train, as she is good fun to be around. The journey this time did not feel so long.

When we arrived, I was way too early to be admitted, so I joined them at their hotel while they booked themselves in. I was automatically jealous of them, as I wished I was booking into the hotel as well. We took it easy for a while and I headed down to get admitted. Again, it did not take too long to get admitted, but instead of having a room to myself, I had to share with other people, which I found a bit uncomfortable to be honest. I had never been used to a hospital environment before until now, and this was a first for me. The people there were nice and I just kept to myself really.

The next morning two nurses came in all gowned-up with their purple gloves. They did the usual double-checking of my vitals and then I was hooked once more onto the chemotherapy drug. I was getting fed up of being stuck on a drip, but if it did the job it was meant to do, then it was worth it.

The next day I felt a bit weak and sick, and when they took the bloods, the readings were not that good. This meant I could not go home. All I wanted to do was cry. My haemoglobin was low, so I had to get two blood transfusions. I wasn`t allowed home until my bloods returned to normal and I didn't handle that very well. I was completely freaked out because, while this was the normal run of events when you were on chemotherapy, this was my first time experiencing it and it spooked me completely. All I wanted to do was go home.

I drove all the nurses mad asking if I could go home every time I saw them, and I just retreated into myself. My Father came up and he ended up having to stay for a night. Thankfully though, on the third extra day, the bloods returned to normal. Professor Carney said that in light of what had happened, I could have an extra few days at home and that I would only be getting half the chemotherapy treatment the next time. Though at that moment this made me happy, it also made me a little paranoid about it as well. Did that mean the chemotherapy was working or was that going to affect the outcome in the long run? So many questions, so many of them that could not be answered.

When I got home I had the usual mouth ulcers and I was sick as normal, but not as bad as last time. The bloods came back normal and I was relieved. I got to see the dogs which uplifted my spirits somewhat. I could now sense the time coming closer to this major surgery and I had an awful feeling I might not make it through. I wished I could talk it through with someone, but I had to be strong for my family and my friends.

It was just Mom and myself that went up to Dublin for the fourth cycle of chemotherapy. I kept thinking that once I got this out of the way, I would have a whole month off. But then looming there was the reality of this major surgery. The fourth cycle of chemotherapy went without a hitch, thank God, and I got home in one piece, delighted with the fact that I was free of chemotherapy for the next few months anyway. I was keeping the surgery well and truly out of my mind for as long as possible. I was sick for a week afterwards with the usual mouth ulcers, but they eventually cleared. My bloods were good, so now I was in the clear and free to recover for the next month.

Surgery

Fatigue was now the biggest obstacle to overcome. Initially, my energy levels were at a low ebb, though slowly, with the help of a good diet, I gradually began to get stronger. I got out to walk the dogs as much as I could, motivated by the fear that I might no longer be able to do so if they had to amputate my leg. My friend Niamh was particularly brilliant, calling over constantly, taking me places and simply just being there for me. I would have been lost without her. At times like this, you really find out who your friends are, and I was fortunate enough to have a great support system of friends.

As I was gaining more strength, I actually started to acquire a new-found interest in cooking. Karen's Mom, bless her, bought me a Delia Smith cookbook and I practiced a few recipes. My confidence grew to the point that I felt ready to organise a dinner party for three of my friends, Karen, Margaret and Niamh. I spent the whole of that day cooking. I was quite proud of myself, having managed to make some brown bread, tomato soup and a fisherman's pie. It took me the whole day and I was wiped out before it had even begun. Yet I was very proud of myself. I think it shocked my friends when they realised that I could cook.

I could feel the time edge ever so closer to that dreaded appointment with Professor Masterson, to discuss my options. Nothing but worry and more worry. Yet when I was at home, it was a default mechanism of mine, to isolate myself inside a bubble of sorts that protected me from the real world. Bad idea I know, but this was my way of coping.

Shane was organising to be home for a few weeks before and after the surgery, and I was looking forward to seeing him and his family. A couple of days before they were due to arrive, I received word that my nephew Patrick had come down with the chicken pox. Unfortunately, that therefore meant that I could not be around them, because it would be too dangerous for me to be exposed to that virus, no matter how long I had been off chemotherapy. Chemotherapy depletes your immune system to such a level that you are susceptible to the slightest infection. I could not afford to get sick now because of the surgery. It hurt me not to be able to spend time with my nephew.

I went to see Professor Masterson, accompanied by Katie, and we discussed my options. It began to look as if amputation was the safer option. This was no simple leg amputation, however, but rather a hind quarter removal, which would take away part of my buttocks as well. This was a major decision. There was around a five per cent chance of it coming back again if I chose amputation and a 10 per cent chance of it recurring if he tried to save my leg, assuming that the tumour could be removed with good margins. How could a person make a decision like that? I had never been good at making any kind of decisions for myself, so this was definitely too much for me to handle. What should I do?

Dr Masterson told me to take a week to consider my options and then return to him in order to make a final decision. My head was wrecked already and I did not have a clue what to do. Of course everyone had an opinion, but this one was mine to make, as I would have to live with this decision. Do I take a chance and live with that 10 per cent chance of it recurring, or do I opt for a lesser chance of it recurring, and in so doing, lose my leg and part of my buttocks? Fitting a prosthesis was going to be difficult because I was already missing some of my buttocks. There was so much to take in and so little time. I did not know what to do.

For most of that week, in my mind, I was being brave and going for the amputation option. Almost too soon it was time to go back down to Professor Masterson, and Shane and Mom came down with me. They were insistent that I should try to save my leg. I thought differently.

My advice for anyone that is in this awful predicament, is that it's a decision not to be made lightly and that, ultimately, it is you and only you that has to make the decision, not your family or your friends. Listen to their opinions, because one way or another they are very much involved with your treatment. But, at the end of the day, it's you that has to live with that decision. Listen to your doctor because he is the one doing the operation, and if he is confident in doing one procedure, it could very well mean saving your limb.

When I got into the room once again, we went over the choices. He could see I was still very unsure and he wanted me to make the right decision. He was not advocating one option above the other. He gave me an hour to decide. I left, with my brother and mother on my tail flying the banner for the leg-saving procedure. I knew their hearts were in the right place, but this was a major decision and I needed to make the right one for me. What could I live with? So I politely told them I wanted some time on my own to be able to think.

I rang Karen, because she has always been a rock

and a very good source of advice to me. I would have been completely lost without her. We talked it through for a while, as I stood there chain-smoking like never before. Mom and Shane found me and told me it was time to go back up. So here we were and I still did not have a clue what to do. Finally, I decided that I was going to throw a question at Professor Masterson, and if I liked the answer I was going to go with that.

When I made it up to the room, we sat down and he looked at me waiting for me to say the word. I asked him what he thought I should do, and if he felt that the tumour could be removed with clear margins. A clear margin means not having to cut too close to the tumour. The closer it is necessary to cut, the higher the risk that cancer cells spread into the blood stream. He looked at me and answered honestly that he could try, and if he thought it too risky then he may have to amputate. Well that sounded good to me. So he was going to try and save the leg and remove the tumour. I took a nervous breath and I silently prayed for this to go right. If this went according to plan, this guy would deserve a very big hug from a very scared and grateful patient. My mother and brother were obviously thrilled with the decision. Funny really what makes us happy when times are really crap!!

The next day I took the dogs for a big long walk in Ballyseedy Woods, feeling that this might be my last walk in these woods for quite some time. It was the nicest of walks, the dogs enjoyed themselves, and yet I could not help feeling sad and apprehensive about the whole situation. Why did this have to happen to me? Stop! I had to stop feeling sorry for myself and show a strong front for the sake of my family. The weekend before the surgery, my two brothers and friends went out with me for a few drinks in Ballybunion. Though the Feale Bar was crowded, we had a lovely night - it felt like my last night of freedom.

On the morning of August 5th, with a very nervous pain in my tummy, I drove Shane and myself to Limerick Regional Hospital. This was it. The reality of hospital administration, however, had to be faced first, and it took an awfully long time to get admitted. I had to go for a series of scans and X-rays and got a blood test. Shane eventually left that evening and I settled in for a sleepless night.

That evening, the anaesthetist came in to see me, and frightened me further by telling me that I was going to be having an epidural, as well as a full anaesthetic. Again, I must stress I had no experience of major operations or anything of the sort, so this was a really scary situation for me. I know I probably did a very good job of appearing to be brave, but this was just a mask to hide the scared child within.

When he left, another doctor came to tell me that I was a very popular person, as everyone wanted in on the operation, as they didn't get to see this type of procedure every day of the week. In a way, I felt flattered and then he told me I was lucky with the type of cancer I had, because there was another one similar to mine, but was faster-growing, and he had a patient who died from it. I was grateful to know that, in a way. He gave me some medication in order to empty my bowels, as this operation was likely to last eight to nine hours.

Following a sleepless night, the nurse arrived early that morning to put on my gown, socks and cap. At 7.50am, Professor Masterson passed by, saw that I was quite nervous, and suggested to the nurse to give me a valium. I was grateful. So at 8am, they wheeled me up to theatre. There was a buzz about the place, nurses preparing instruments, hooking me onto monitors and organising the epidural. After that, all was a blur...

I opened my eyes slowly. I was in the ICU and extremely groggy. It was dark and I could tell it was late at night. I felt very thirsty and I had a grumpy male nurse who obliged with one of those sponge pops soaked with water. But it was not enough. I wanted more. He wouldn't, however, allow me anymore, afraid perhaps that I would get sick. I could not move and I was slowly becoming more aware of where I was and what was happening. I went in and out of consciousness for most of the night and I did not look down to see whether I had a leg or not. I was afraid to. I was also hooked onto central lines and all kinds of monitors.

When I awoke again it was morning and my mother and father were there. They looked pleased to see me awake and there was also a big fruit basket from work, wishing me well. I didn`t ask them anything and then the one person I wanted to see came in - Professor Masterson. He had a big smile and I thought, 'Well, this has to be good. Fingers crossed!' He said the operation was a success, he had gotten good margins and he had saved my leg. He also told me that the size of the tumour was roughly the size of my head. Apparently, at one stage of the operation, my leg was totally detached from my body apart from some muscle and nerves. I was so relieved, I gave him a big hug and thanked him. I had to stay in the ICU for a day or two, as I still had the epidural in place in order to keep the pelvis very still so that it could heal.

After a day or two, they removed the central lines and I only had a normal drip by the time I got down to my room. It was good to be out of the ICU, though frustration immediately followed, as I was longing to get outside for a cigarette. I was not allowed to leave the bed until physio cleared me. Eventually they came, and they had to show me the safe and correct way of getting out of bed, as well as showing me how to walk using a Zimmer frame. The pain, when getting out of bed, was of a level that I have never before experienced, and therefore all I could manage was a mere few steps. It was agony, but it was worth it, as they brought out a wheelchair and my mother was able to wheel me downstairs and out for a cigarette.

I believed now that my addiction to smoking provided me with an incentive to get up and break through the pain barrier, an incentive I would not have had had I not smoked at the time. When I got back to the room it was nearly worse getting back into the bed. I didn't think this recovery was going to be easy. I was hooked onto a catheter and had a lot of stitches. The physio came every day. They planned for me to be moved down to Croom Hospital for recuperation and rehabilitation, but I developed an infection which prevented me from going there.

I had to get surgery done once a week to clean out the wound and it was really annoying as I had to be last on the list for theatre because of the infection. I had to fast from midnight the night before, for a procedure that normally occurred at 3 or 4 pm.

After a week or two the stitches were out, and the wound where the infection was located had a vac

45

pump attached. This is a brilliant device that sucks all the pus and detritus from the wound, promoting a faster healing. So now I had another attachment. I was on a drip to get antibiotics each evening and the physio said I was doing so well that I could start using crutches, but because of the drip line in my hand I could not. Friends from work were very good and called in to see me. Clare was very good and came most mornings to wheel me out for my morning cigarette. Things were progressing slowly.

I was there nearly a month at this stage, and I was really starting to want to go home. I heard from one of the nurses that if they saw me walking more, then perhaps there was a chance that I would be discharged. So I started walking down for my cigarette. The only thing that was slowing things up at this stage was the infection. I still had to go down to theatre to get the wound cleaned out. It was now six weeks that I had been in hospital. One day, I was sitting outside and I saw someone walking their dog, and that was it, I had had enough. I wanted to go home. I missed my dogs and I was starting to get really fed up.

So the next day, when I saw Professor Masterson, I asked him. He said that once I could tolerate having the wound cleaned without the use of a strong sedative, then I could go home on the Monday, because they had to organise the district nurse to call to the house to clean the wound every two days or so. I was very nervous over the cleaning of the wound, because I was not great with things like that. Friday came, and in the afternoon the nurse came in and gave me a painkiller and this pop to suck on that was also a painkiller. The doctors came in and they started. It was not that bad at all, a little uncomfortable, but tolerable. I was delighted by my body's reaction as it meant that I could now go home on Monday!

So on Monday afternoon, Katie came and collected me. I said goodbye to all my favourite nurses and off I went on my crutches. The journey home was not that bad and I was just excited to get home and see the house again. To have my bed back again was a great feeling of triumph. My first night was lovely. I had a very peaceful night's sleep and I was to meet the district nurse the following day for the first time. The thoughts of changing my bandages made me nervous again, as I was afraid it might hurt more now that I was out of the hospital environment.

At around 10.30am she arrived and got straight down to business. The wound took a while to clean as the dressing and then the sponge (that was in the wound with a tube attached to suck out the bad pus), had to be removed. Then the wound had to be cleaned, and another sponge, the same size as the wound, was inserted back in and the pump reattached and redressed. It all took approximately a half hour to an hour. The district nurses came every second day to clean the wound.

On the second week of being home, I had to go up to see Professor Masterson in his outpatients' clinic. He was happy with the way the wound was healing and said it was going to take a bit of time to fully heal. So I went to Limerick every two weeks and I was doing a lot of walking with the crutches. My leg began to feel much stronger. I was also becoming more active. The wound was getting much smaller and when I went to see Professor Masterson in Croom he decided that it could be stitched up. So he stitched it up and he said that hopefully, within the next two weeks, it should have fully closed up.

It was now coming towards the end of September and I could not believe how the time had flown, and yet, how long it had taken the wound to heal. So in the next few weeks, I could be going back on the chemotherapy. A feeling of doom enveloped me. I then got an appointment with a physio in Listowel and Katie took me in. When I was there I was not that happy, as she was giving me exercises to do at home – anyone that knows me knows that I just don`t do homework!!! My leg was much stronger and I felt like I was ready to go onto one crutch, but was not sure how to do that myself. I did not want to take any unnecessary risks.

Friends from work came up to see me one weekend and we went to Tralee for coffee. We were outside talking for a while and whatever way I was leaning on my crutches caused me to fall. I was instantly petrified, praying that I had not done any major damage. Someone helped me up and I went back in with a very sore ego!! All the girls were very concerned about me but I was grand. When I got home, I thought about what had happened, and I decided to go into casualty to have my leg X-rayed, just in case. It would never do to have a setback now. So when I got in, they were very good, and I got down to be X-rayed without any major delay. The doctor then had a look and, thankfully, there was no damage to the hip. The next week I was back down to see Professor Masterson and the wound was now fully healed, so now it was back to Professor Carney for more chemotherapy. What fun!

More Chemotherapy

Physiotherapy treatment left me a little underwhelmed, so I decided to forego it until I finished with the chemotherapy, as I was going to be too knackered and sick anyway. My appointment to see Professor Carney was scheduled for the following week, but I let my mother talk me into ringing him and having the consult over the phone, because she was overly-concerned about me having to travel all the way up to Dublin, even though I would have to do so when I started chemotherapy again. He was very understanding though, unfortunately, he had to inform me that the chemotherapy that I was on did not really work for me, as when they tested the tumour that was removed, there was not much evidence of dead cancer cells and, furthermore, the tumour had not really reduced in size. Not exactly what I was hoping to hear.

So, I was now going to try a different chemotherapy drug, which was to be administered for a longer time than previously - 12 hours straight for five days straight. It had to take place in Dublin, but there was no way I could afford to stay in the Mater

Private. I told him that I would have to go to the Mater Public this time, and he said he would have to get back to me as to when it was going to happen, because he was not sure whether or not there would be a bed available in the next week or two. That was fine with me, because it gave me time to prepare mentally as well as physically. I could not believe I was at this stage of the treatment cycle. It has gone so fast, yet so slow. I felt like my life had stopped and I didn`t know if I would ever be able to pick up the pieces of my previous life. I could handle all the surgeries in the world, it was the chemotherapy and going to Dublin that was really hard to deal with. I didn`t think I would ever be able to go to Dublin again after this.

It was now mid-November, and my cat Mojo had been missing for the past few days. He suddenly reappeared very sick and, typically, on a Sunday. To make things even worse, the road was closed due to some car rally going on, so I tried to keep the cat hydrated as much as possible. In the early afternoon, while I was preparing dinner with my mother, my mobile rang. Strange, a Dublin number coming up. I answered the phone to find out it was the Mater Public hospital saying there was a bed free and that I was to come in straight away. My brain froze. I could not think for a second. I had been expecting to hear from Professor Carney beforehand. I guess not. I told them my predicament of the road being closed, but they said to come up today or the bed could be gone by the next day. So that was the end of my dinner. I could not eat a thing.

The first thing I did was to ring Karen to see whether she would be able to take the dogs at such short notice, I was packing as I was talking to her. We were both in shock. Nausea enveloped me, exacerbated by the fact that I had no time to mentally prepare for this. So we decided that Dad would take me up, and Mom would get the train on Tuesday morning, as she needed to stay with the dogs and pack herself. So I rang the vet on call and asked could I bring the cat in on our way to Dublin. Once that was organised we had to check with the guards about getting on the road. Luckily, by the time I got myself and my stuff together, the rally was more or less finished.

We got on the road, making a pit stop at the vets in Listowel. The trip to Dublin was long, lengthened by the fact that I really just wanted to turn around and go home and hide under the bed and pretend it was not happening. I tried to pull myself together. If I did not go through with this I was going to get the cancer back again and I could die. I gave myself that pep-talk all the way up to Dublin. Once again, I felt all alone. There was not a sinner who could rescue me. Would I ever see the light? Would I ever get my life back on

53

track? Questions to which I never really expected to hear an answer.

When we entered the hospital it seemed both very big and very scary. I was sent up to an oncology ward, sharing a room with five others, with just one TV between us. I could already tell this was going to be a long week. I told my father to leave as he had a four-hour journey ahead of him. So we said our goodbyes. I settled in for the night, or tried to anyway. My head was not in this at all, I hate change and I hated the way this happened so suddenly. I like to know what awaits me so that I have time to prepare. I was out of my depth again and I did not like it.

The next morning I found out that my port channel was not drawing any blood, so they had to find a vein in order to start the chemotherapy. Later on that day, I was then sent down to get it X-rayed, to ensure that the port was in the vein in order for it to be used to administer the chemotherapy drug. Thankfully it was. It was strange being in this hospital, as I did not know any of the nurses. I also found that getting out to have a cigarette was an extremely laborious process, as I had a drip stand and a wheelchair to contend with, not to mention the big long walk. I appreciate that smoking is very bad for you, particularly considering the disease I have, but patients have rights and they have a right to smoke if they please, and the HSE and the government should not make it impossible for patients to have a cigarette, particularly those that have walking difficulties.

I didn`t see Professor Carney until Tuesday morning, and by then chemotherapy had started. I had not really started to feel any serious side-effects yet. I was glad my mother was coming later that day because it would be easier to get out for a cigarette, even though one the doctors did not approve. Some of the nurses seemed nice, but you could not help but sense the level of pressure they were under. I did not really strike up any relationship with any of them, not like the ones I built up with the nurses in the Mater Private anyway. The high volume of patients coming through the doors of public hospitals means that forming any kind of patient relationship is simply an impossibility.

Mom was here now and it was great my arm was not sore from trying to push myself on the wheelchair and managing the drip stand as well. At this stage, I was managing to walk with one crutch and carry the drip stand to the toilet. The last time I had to do this was before my operation, when both my legs were fully functional. They wanted me to pee into a jug so they had a good idea of how much I was drinking and how much I was excreting, in order to ensure my kidneys were functioning correctly. I found it hard anyway.

On Thursday, I missed Professor Carney's rounds that morning, and the other doctors were not pleased that I had missed him. One female doctor, in particular, really upset me, because she did not want me leaving the ward to go anywhere, not to mind outside for a cigarette. I did not like this hospital. It felt far too impersonal. I felt totally alone and the staff were merely going through the motions. I appreciate they were probably run off their feet, but from my personal patient point of view, I was receiving merely mediocre care.

Today was Friday and I was looking forward to the next day, because I was going to be going home once chemotherapy was finished in the afternoon and the bloods were OK. It had not been that bad this time really. I only felt sick once, however, I was feeling very fatigued. I was hopeful. I was told that the immunity could get really low with this type of chemotherapy, so I had be really careful in terms of the people I came in contact with. I had to discuss the dogs with Karen, and we both agreed that she would hold onto them until I got my bloods done, and once my immunity levels recovered, I could get them back.

I was now going to have a three-week break, which was not that bad. That evening dragged, as well as the following morning. Time felt like as if it was not moving fast enough. I was really looking forward to getting home. We planned to get the train down to Limerick and my brother Aidan was to collect us from there and drive us home. It was the afternoon by the time they came around and said the bloods were good and that I was able to go home. The relief was indescribable, as I really did not want to spend another minute there. A relative had heard about the week that I had spent in the public hospital and offered to cover the cost of going to the Mater Private next time. I was deeply grateful as I really did not want to go back there.

The journey down on the train was OK; it was a little bit awkward because of the wheelchair and the entire luggage. However, the staff were brilliant and very helpful. It's funny the way people treat you when they see you in a wheelchair. Some pretend not to see you at all, some look on you with pity and some were curious. I began to acquire a new respect for people with walking difficulties. I could now see how they were treated.

When we arrived in Limerick, my brother Aidan was waiting for us, and it was not long before we were on the road back to Kerry. We talked about work as we both worked for the same company. I found that I missed my colleagues and the work, and wished I was back there. If I ever got back to work, I was never going to take it for granted again. After an hour and a half, we arrived home and it was good to be back. I felt extremely tired, though not tired enough to check my temperature before going to bed. Thankfully it was good.

On Tuesday evening, I was doing my usual temperature check, a little worried that my temperature was up. I decided to give it half an hour before checking it again and then to decide what to do from there. After a half an hour passed, I checked my temperature again and it had indeed risen slightly from the level of before. So I called my mother and told her to ring the Mater Private to see what advice they had to offer. They instructed me to check it in an hour, and if it was still up, to go to the nearest casualty. So we waited on tenterhooks. I still felt hot and I sensed that my temperature was not likely to come down at all. An hour later I stuck the thermometer in my mouth and waited for the beep. It felt like the longest time ever. When I took it out my temperature was still up. So I got up and dressed, feeling guilty at the same time, because I was causing all this trouble. I was causing my mother all this stress which must not be good for her.

My father drove us into the hospital. I was wondering how long this was going to take as I was not feeling that bad, and I really preferred being back at home. So when I came into casualty, I explained to the woman that I was undergoing chemotherapy treatment in Dublin and that they had advised me to check in at the nearest casualty, as my temperature was up. So she led me straight away to a triage nurse who proceeded to check my blood pressure and my temperature again. My temperature had now risen appreciably to 39 degrees.

Whilst undergoing chemotherapy treatment the use of paracetamol is prohibited, therefore, when your temperature rises, it is important to be seen by a doctor. The nurse sent me to a room on my own and said that she would get a doctor, as well as having someone come to take my bloods. I was very impressed. Here I was, thinking that it would be hours before I was seen, and all I had to do now was to see the doctor and get bloods and hopefully all would be OK.

So the nurse came in and tried to take some blood. I warned her that I had difficult veins and sure enough she was having no luck. In the end she had to call an anaesthetist to take the bloods. They were checking my temperature, while I was waiting for my results. They were worried that the underlying cause of the rise in my temperature was an infection. I made sure that they knew I was not allowed to take paracetamol. The weather outside was freezing, so it was not so nice going out for a cigarette.

After an hour, the doctor came in to confirm that I did indeed have an infection and that, therefore, I had to stay in hospital for the week to be put on IV antibiotics. I looked at him in disbelief. At least I was in Tralee, which made it easier for my family, and it was my first time staying in Kerry General Hospital. I was impressed from the off by their A&E unit. The staff were all so nice and welcoming and it was such a change from Dublin. So, once again, I was hooked onto a drip with that gnawing sense of being tied down. I sent both Mom and Dad home for the night, as outside the weather was getting colder. Severe frosts were forecast. When I looked outside the window it seemed as if it was already freezing. I wish I was at home.

My Consultant visited on rounds the next morning and said that my temperature was still up and that if it got any higher they would have to give me paracetamol. He also informed me they were in communication with Professor Carney. My mother came in with stuff and I was distracting myself on the Nintendo.

On Tuesday I started to lose my hair. Nothing prepared me for the loss of dignity I experienced in having to endure this in public. I think perhaps in some ways it was the toughest thing I had to deal with thus far, as I was not at all prepared for it. While I was expecting to lose it, I thought I would be at home on my own and I would not have to have people around me to witness it happening or taking pity on me. I got my Mom to organise a hairdresser to come as I was going to shave the rest off. I was not going to let this get the better of me. I was embarrassed though by the amount of shed hair upon the bed and around the room. So the hairdresser came, and with her went my remaining hair. I looked really weird without any hair. I felt a number of emotions, but again I had to show a strong front for my family's sake.

I was very impressed with the staff of Kerry General and the hospital itself, which was very clean and well run, and it made me wish I was being treated down here. As the week went by, my temperature started to ever so slowly come down, and I thought I would be going home once I was finished with the antibiotics. When I was talking to my consultant on Thursday morning, he said he wanted to keep me in until Sunday and then I was to be transported up to Dublin by ambulance, as the weather was getting worse with frost and snow. He also said I could go home in the early afternoon, but to be back in the hospital for about 8pm so I could finish off the antibiotics. I was fiercely frustrated by the fact that there would be no reprieve from this endless cycle of hospitals and drips.

So that afternoon was great when I got to go home for a few hours. I wasted it watching TV as there was nothing else to do. We had to drive carefully back in that evening as it was quite frosty. Once I got in, I got hooked back on the drip and took it easy for the evening. Niamh called in and surprised me with a Big Mac from McDonald's, which made a nice break from hospital food!!!

The next day when I got home, I got stuff together for the trip back up to Dublin. I was still depressed and found it hard not to show it. It was eventually time to be getting back to the hospital. All the family called to see me the day before, as I would be gone for another week. I did not really want to leave. If I could I would stay in Kerry General. So the following day arrived and I was stretchered into the ambulance and strapped in, which was all very strange. The two paramedics were from Dublin and they were lovely. As we drove up the country the weather was worse in places - foggy, snowing and freezing. Of course I was dying for a cigarette, but now had to wait until we arrived before I would be able to have one. The one consoling thought was that I was going back to the Mater Private rather than the Public!

We eventually arrived and I got out and sat in the freezing cold on the wheelchair to have that long-awaited cigarette. I was so relieved to have the journey over with, but I was still depressed over the whole situation. I decided to ask Professor Carney if I could get the rest of the chemotherapy treatment done down in Kerry General. The next morning I had to get X-rayed again, to make sure the port channel was in place, as it still was not working for drawing up blood. Thankfully, it was still in place, so they hooked me back up and I was once more back on the chemotherapy. This time I was in a room on my own and I was happier because I could watch what I liked on TV and I did not have to disturb anyone else. I brought up my portable DVD player so it was nice to be able to watch a DVD whenever I liked.

The next morning, when Professor Carney was doing his rounds, I worked up the courage to ask him about having the chemotherapy done down in Kerry. He immediately ruled out the possibility due to the extreme type of chemotherapy that I was on. I was disgusted but yet I understood why. The days passed a bit quicker this time thanks to DVDs and the Nintendo. On Friday evening, I was told I had to organise my local surgery nurse to give me an injection, which helps with my immunity, when I was back home on Sunday. I was thankful when it came to Saturday and the blood results came back nice and clear. I was a little nervous going home and I suppose I was also afraid that I would have to go back into hospital again.

All I wanted was to go home, sleep in my own bed and eventually get to see my dogs, as it had been nearly four weeks since I last saw them.

My father collected me as I was not going to take any chances with trains this time. No point in needlessly risking infection. The journey down was tiring and non-eventful. When we got home I checked my temperature and went straight to bed. As it was a Saturday night I watched a bit of TV and fell asleep. The next morning the surgery nurse was scheduled to come at around 12.30pm. So I rested in bed until she came. She was very good and gave me an injection into the belly. I was keeping my fingers and toes crossed that this treatment would work and that no bad infection would visit me. Again, the side-effects to this chemotherapy were not all that bad, as I was not that sick with it, just very tired. It seemed to affect my immunity levels more than anything, which can of course be very dangerous if you're not being careful, but boy did I plan to be. I was determined not to see a hospital until the next trip to Dublin. I just realised I had two more cycles of chemotherapy left and then, with the help of God, I would be finished and I would never have to go through that again. Oh, I was so hopeful that would be the case.

The weather outside was frightful and I was thankful I was inside, nice and warm tucked up in bed, playing the play station 3. Anything to keep the boredom away. The next two days seemed to drift by and so far so good. On Tuesday my temperature was good and I got up for a bit. I went on Facebook for a while and ordered some Christmas presents on Amazon for the nieces and nephews. It was really satisfying that I did not even have to leave the house to shop. How great technology is really. I started to get tired, so I went down early to bed. It was now the 14th of December 2010.

The Pain

After a couple of hours in bed, I woke up with a niggling pain in my bum. It was causing me some discomfort, and try as I might, I could not get comfortable. I checked my temperature to make sure I was not running an infection and fortunately my temperature seemed normal. This same sensation remained for a few hours. By midnight, however, I was in more pain and even more uncomfortable, so I called out to my mother and asked her in a very calm voice to ring the on-call doctor. Being asked endless questions over the phone when you are in pain is the last thing anyone would want, and therefore I was not in the mood for waiting around too long. I was at a loss to know what was causing the pain. All I knew was that it was gradually getting worse.

Eventually the phone rang to inform me that a doctor would be calling within an hour or two. I laughed hysterically as I needed a painkiller fast!! The pain was coming and going with very little intervals of subsidence. By 2am the doctor eventually showed up. He did not examine my bum, but I told him my history and explained the pain, and he gave me a painkiller by injection, saying that if the pain came back again to call. I was slightly annoyed, as I would have preferred to have some explanation of this pain. Most of all though I was hoping that it would never come back again. All that was going through my head was thanking God he did not send me into hospital!!!

The injection lasted for a few hours but by 6am the pain was back again, this time with extreme vengeance. Ebbing and flowing but acquiring momentum by the minute. It was now becoming unbearable. So at 8am my mother called Dr. O'Reilly and, by some chance, got through to him. He came straight away and this time he examined me, but there was no obvious signs of any source of what was causing the pain, so he gave me another painkiller and said if it came back to call him again. I was really getting frustrated and tired at this stage, having spent the night in extreme pain. This time the painkiller did not really work and the pain continued to worsen.

By some miracle the district nurse called in to see me and Mom told her what was happening. She had a look at my bum and immediately called the GP to come down as fast as she could. A red spot had appeared on my buttocks which was causing her great concern. By this stage I was more or less crying with pain. I remember insisting that I was not going into hospital. After five minutes, the doctor arrived, very swiftly had a look at my bum and the next minute she was on the phone calling an ambulance. I was hysterical as I did not want to go back to hospital, in spite of the serious amount of pain I was in. Things started to fade now from my memory. I can remember the ambulance arriving and me being stretchered into the ambulance and me moaning in pain all the way into Tralee. I can remember my mother telling me that the sirens were sounding just for me. I could not take it all in because at this stage the pain was unbearable and then… oblivion.

Contribution from Shane O'Neill
on behalf of the family

A roller coaster ride. That was the metaphor most commonly used during the first month of Ciara's coma and it is perhaps the most apt. For comas are a confusing business. Where once there was the person you knew, there is now that person and a machine. For that person you love would not be alive before your eyes were it not for a machine.

Comas prompt endless questioning. The first and most elemental one concerns the soul itself. Is the person that you have known all your life still alive?

How can that be so if a machine has taken over the breathing function for them? If the body can't breathe itself then is that life force called the soul still there? Such metaphysical questions rise to the surface amidst a clamour of other thoughts and fade away almost as quickly as they arose. For in the end one is so eternally grateful to this machine, because were it not for the machine…The human capacity to create and innovate and in this case, assist nature, humbles you completely.

As we sat night after night with Ciara, the regular electronic ticking of the machine became the sound of her breathing, the lines that were mapped across a computer screen for heart rate and blood pressure became her words. As long as the sounds remained steady and the lines straight then all was somehow ok. This deceiving sense of comfort was often pulled like a pillow from under our lightly dozing heads when the machine began to bleep out a warning sound. Almost immediately a nurse would appear to assure us that it was just an electronic glitch and nothing to worry about. Mollified though nevertheless still tense, for it felt at these moments that Ciara was trying to communicate something.

We read Ciara's progress through these lines in front of us on a computer screen. Lines we did not even properly understand. When things took occasional turns for the worse the symmetry of the lines became messed up and the numbers recording heartbeat, temperature and blood pressure also took on an alarming appearance. Nothing for it but to hold her hand and watch that screen willing the lines and numbers to come good. Steady lines and steady numbers meant somehow that her body was getting a chance in the background to come back from wherever it was.

Small signs of progress would be made over the course of a number of days and it became easy to be fooled into an idea of progression. That this all followed a straight line somehow. Due to the severe nature of Ciara's wound, the level of pain she was enduring and the detrimental effects of intense chemotherapy upon her body's defenses, progress was never likely to follow a straight line. Rather it followed the proverbial roller coaster taking our emotions and the staffs' emotions for a ride with it. The sheer horror of this moment we were all living with her was further complicated by the fact that her kidneys were failing. Toxic byproducts were building up in her body and likely to put her kidneys in extreme danger. So not only was she in a coma induced state but now there was an imminent possibility that she would have to be transferred to another hospital that provided dialysis support for ICU patients. Thankfully however this did not come to pass.

Instead Ciara struggled on, in the end spending almost seven weeks in the Intensive Care Unit. All that we could do was hold her hand, read to her occasionally and maintain a physical presence in case she one day miraculously woke up. If you are of a positive disposition then you naturally believe that this will happen, if you tend to be of a more pessimistic persuasion then you begin to feel foolish talking to a person who is never likely to hear you. Most of us are, I think, an endlessly shifting mix of the two, riding on that rollercoaster, feeling one moment that all will be well with our loved one and another moment feeling that we will never see them again. Miraculously it became possible to wake Ciara from her induced coma as her body's natural defenses were finally revived. Her family are still conscious to this day that a machine kept her alive for long enough to summon home those troops to fight on her behalf. She went on to make a full recovery.

Ciara feels it is important to portray the coma experience from a family viewpoint. In the end though what we all thought and experienced didn't seem important anymore, for she was coming back to us and appeared to be getting better. And this was all that mattered.

A note from Mr. John Rice

Orthopaedic Surgeon

I first met Ciara when she was brought by ambulance to the Emergency Department on 15/12/10. Ciara was in severe pain at the time of admission and she had an area of cellulitis/abscess formation in her left buttock. Our initial concern was Ciara`s level of pain and we treated her with opioid analgesia. She was admitted to hospital however, shortly after admission it became apparent that Ciara had systemic sepsis and was developing septic shock, a condition whereby her heart rate increased and her blood pressure decreased due to the toxins in her blood stream. Ciara was barely conscious at that stage and my initial communication was with her mother Peggy rather than Ciara herself due to the extent of her pain and her generalized weakness. Ciara responded well to her initial treatment of intravenous antibiotics and intravenous fluids. She was transferred to the Intensive Care Unit and required inotropic support to maintain her blood pressure.

She was brought to the Operating Theatre the following day on 16/12/10. At that stage, we incised an abscess and an area of cellulitis in her left buttock and applied a vacuum dressing. Ciara remained on

73

intravenous fluid and was maintained on ventolin support in the Intensive Care Unit. We were concerned about Ciara`s wellbeing at that stage and I discussed her case with both Prof. Masterson in Limerick and Prof. Des Carney in the Mater in Dublin and both of these doctors encouraged us to pursue an aggressive line in terms of her medical management. as they felt that if she came over the septic shock that occurred as a complication of her chemotherapy for her Osteosarcoma, that she would do well.

Over the next few days, I became actively involved in her Intensive Care Unit Management Consultation with the Anaesthetist in Kerry General Hospital. Her condition remained critical and I recall having in-depth conversation with her parents and brother Shane in relation to her survival. I clearly recall a conversation with her mother at that stage when Ciara`s lungs, kidney`s and liver were not functioning due to the overwhelming sepsis. Peggy seemed to have a deep rooted faith and we both agreed that in the Intensive Care Unit we would support Ciara in terms of her respiratory function and in terms of providing fluid and antibiotics, but the rest we would leave to God. We then entered the Christmas period and Ciara continued to be ventilated and could not communicate with her family or with the medical staff looking after her.

74

On 23/12/2010, we brought her to the Operating Theatre and carried out radical surgery excising a lot of the dead and infected tissue in the region of her left buttocks. We managed her wound using a vacuum dressing. This posed a significant challenge for us to get a feel on this dressing to lower continuous suction to encourage healing at the wound. Her wound management was further complicated by the fact that she had a bleeding disorder due to her sepsis and the vacuum dressing frequently filled with blood. We however, persisted with aggressive intensive care unit management and we recognised that while it appeared that she had kidney failure a lot of the increase in her urea and creatinine was due to lack of protein in the blood. We instigated nasal gastric feeding initially, but this was not successful however, on the 29/12/2010 we were to bring her back to the Operating Theatre and site a feeding tube in her jejunum or small bowel. This permitted us to get a high volume of high protein fluid into her small bowel to help to aid healing. We carried out further debridements of her infected tissue in her left buttock and we saw a gradual improvement in Ciara`s form over the next three weeks. Ciara remained unconscious in the Intensive Care Unit and management of her bowel function become a problem due to proximity of her bowel to the large wound in her left buttock. We therefore arranged with Mr Kevin Murray that Ciara would undergo a colectomy to divert faeces into a colostomy bag on her abdomen and to keep it away from the area of the wound. Ciara`s form improved dramatically over the next two weeks. I recall at that stage, photographs of her dogs were brought into the single room in the Operating Theatre and Ciara got fantastic family support, they continued to talk to Ciara even though she was unconscious and had an endotracheal tube in her upper airway. This tube prevented her from talking however, this tube was removed at the end of January 2011 and a tracheostomy tube was placed in her neck that allowed her to breath by herself.

Ciara was discharged from the Intensive Care Unit on 07/01/2011 and transferred to Clonfert ward. Over the next few weeks, her form and ability to walk around improved dramatically and it was only at this stage that I first began to talk to Ciara and to get to know her as a person. She still had a large wound in her buttock, but towards the end of February 2011 she begun to make incredible strides and by the 25/02/2011 we found it difficult to keep Ciara in hospital. She was discharged home and the arrangement initially was that she would come to see us on a weekly basis for attention to her vacuum dressing in the Outpatients Department. She had a short admission in the middle of March 2011 when we carried out skin grafting of the wound in her buttocks, but physically and psychologically Ciara thrived over the next three months.

The Long Road to Recovery

I cannot quite remember the very first time I awoke, but I certainly remember the groggy sensation. I also remember being conscious of the fact that I was heavily medicated. I, however, did not know who I was never mind where I was, though I was conscious of my mother being in the room. I also could not talk. I fell back asleep again. When I woke up again, I realised that I was in a hospital bed and connected to all kinds of monitors. I could barely move my hands as they felt so heavy. I asked Mum what had happened but my voice was barely audible. I felt something scratchy at my throat and was not sure what it was. My mother looked very relieved. I was wondering why. What happened? Memory was not running back to its owner as quickly as its owner would have liked.

My mother tried to soothe me, saying that I was in the ICU, and the reason I could not talk was because I was hooked up to a ventilator for the last couple of weeks. What couple of weeks? What did she mean? What the hell happened? She then said something and I felt that I had not heard correctly. She repeated it again, saying that it was the middle of January and I had missed the whole of Christmas and all the New Year. I could not take this in; my mind went numb with shock. All I could remember was the ambulance ride into hospital. Nurses were coming and going taking care of all the tubes and wires I was hooked up to. Then they mentioned something about a wound and how extreme it was. What the hell had happened to me? I looked down at my hands and I could see they were quite swollen. I tried writing what I wanted to ask but my writing was totally illegible.

For those first few days I was in and out of sleep. My leg felt worse than before and I was really confused. I later found out that I had nearly died. The information filtered very slowly through to me. I could not take much in anyway, as I was still too drugged up. When I became slightly more aware, I was told I had an abscess which had burst and when I got to A&E, I was completely neutropenic, which meant my immunity was non-existent. I succumbed to septicemia and they mentioned something about my kidneys having nearly failed. It felt like someone had rolled over me with all that news. I still could not believe it.

I was still very weak and I was still using oxygen. I had a gastric tube in place in order to be tube-fed. I also had this thing called an emergency colostomy in place, which at the time meant nothing to me. I realised they had to operate on my bum where the abscess was and that the wound was big. That's all I knew for now. I had no co-ordination. I could not get out of bed, and to all intents and purposes, I was like a vegetable.

As the days began to pass, my voice was slowly getting a little bit stronger and my writing was slightly improving. Niamh came in one day with sponge balls and I could not even throw them. I could tell the family were all very relieved though, and sensed that they had been through some kind of hell and back while I was lying in my hospital bed. That stressed me out because I did not want them under any kind of stress over me. The nurses were constantly coming in and out, and I had to get my wound cleaned regularly which I did not like, as it was very sore. Despite my many requests, no-one would take a picture for me to see it.

I was still in the ICU, though I was beginning to get a bit stronger each day. They eventually hoisted me out of bed but it was ever so painful, although I did manage to get outside for a cigarette! The physio was very nice and understanding. I was still extremely weak but the hospital porters seemed happy to wheel me out, in order to satisfy my cravings. I could not even light it up as the power in my hands was still minimal. The task was further complicated by the significant shake I now had in my hands, which was supposedly a side-effect of the massive quantities of morphine I had been on. Something like morphine withdrawal symptoms. I then had to be hoisted back into bed. It hurt but it was worth it. I was so absolutely knackered after that first trip, that I slept most of that evening.

My voice was getting much stronger but I still needed the oxygen some evenings. I still used the food tube and I started to eat very small amounts at a time. I also had to drink this blue water which was supposed to have beneficial effects on my kidneys. I also still had the catheter in place. As the weeks went by, I was getting a little bit stronger. I hated the dressing changes. It hurt like hell but the nurses from the ICU had a special knack which did not make it that bad. I was in and out of surgery to clean the wound and I was still very tired and very much out of it. My mother was great, she was in and out to see me every day, but I could see the effects the last few months had on her, which really worried me. The staff were all brilliant and all very supportive, from the nurses to cleaners and canteen staff.

At this stage, they removed the peg feed tube from my throat as I was no longer using the ventilator, and I suppose they saw me as being out of the woods. My voice was getting a bit better, yet I remained very hoarse. I was still in a state of disbelief over what had happened. Try as I might, I could not quite process that I had nearly died, how lucky I was to still be here and how I had missed the whole of Christmas and the New Year.

Mom had been singing the praises of a consultant called Mr. Rice, saying how brilliant he was and how he had saved my life. I had yet to meet him. At first, I was wary because this was another doctor on the scene, one I did not know. I would have to see and find out for myself. If I had met him already, I could not recall. My memory was still a bit hazy from all the drugs. In total, I had spent seven weeks in the ICU before I was transferred to another ward. When I was told I was being moved, I did not really like that idea, as I knew all the nurses and I was more comfortable being there. But the porters came in and playfully reprimanded me, saying that I should be delighted because this meant that I was not in any serious danger and I did not need to be there holding up a bed.

So when I got to Clonfert Ward, it took me a while to adjust. When it came to the dress change, I wanted the nurses from the ICU, and thankfully they obliged. I will always be ever so grateful to the nurses of Kerry General. They keep that hospital ticking and they are simply extremely dedicated, professional and caring individuals. They all deserve medals in my eyes.

The next morning Mr. Rice was doing his rounds. He was a young guy and seemed very down to earth. He did not seem like your typical consultant and he was very understanding. He discussed what was happening and he knew I was not really taking much in, as I was still on a good deal of medication and my concentration levels were negligible. I was slowly being weaned off morphine over the last few weeks and my hands were constantly shaking. Hallucinations visited me every hour.

It was now February and I was much stronger, well when I say stronger I mean I had made small little bits of improvement. I was far from being 100 per cent, nor did I ever think that I would be. My leg was useless. I was told that I had lost a lot of muscle which had completely weakened my leg. I had to go down to the Physio department to see Finn each day and it was really hard work because he had me walking up and down a gymnasium floor using a Zimmer frame. It hurt like hell and I was actually out of breath after doing one length of the room. I had absolutely no energy but he pushed me to keep going as much as I could.

Mid-February came and I was really starting to miss my dogs and home, so when Mr. Rice was doing his rounds, I begged him to let me go home. I could see that he was not very comfortable with the idea because of the size of the wound, plus I was some

84

distance from being better. But I could see that he was tempted to concede to my wishes. So any time I saw him, I asked if I could go home and eventually he did give in, allowing me home under very strict instructions. We also tried the vac pump on the wound, the same one I had following my tumour removal. He was hoping that it would work and help accelerate the healing process. The wound was still both very extensive and very deep. I gave him a big hug because I was so relieved and grateful, but also because I could see he was still a bit uncomfortable with the idea. My mother also had a big job in front of her, as she was going to be taking care of me. I would already have been lost without her. I had been in hospital for two months straight. As a parting word, Mr. Rice requested that I come to visit his Outpatients Clinic once a week, and also mentioned that I may have to come back into hospital to get the wound cleaned. Also if the vac pump did not work, an alternative plan had to be thought of to promote better healing. I had to organise the district nurses as well. I was so grateful and excited to be going home that I was barely listening.

When I got home, an electronic hospital bed had been ordered for me. This was a wonderful help as it had a motorised elevation function that would help me to raise myself in bed. The district nurse was to call every day. I was still heavily medicated for the pain, the raw nerves, and I cannot tell for what else. That first week passed in a blur. The vac pump was constantly giving trouble, as the size of my wound was so big that it kept losing suction. It was quite annoying because every time it lost suction, an alarm would go off which had to be reset in order to silence it. One night, it kept the whole house awake. Another night, a particularly vicious cramp in my leg kept me awake and in tears. It was a horrible ordeal, one that I did not think would ever end. Once I got rid of one pain, another one arose from somewhere else. It never once subsided and it was most definitely my worst best friend at that moment. It also had everyone around me tormented.

Wednesday arrived quickly and it was time for me to see the consultant again. Not that I was processing that much information. I was basically living inside of myself a lot of the time and my body was just going, or barely going, to where it needed to. My mother seemed to trust him and like him though, so that would have to do for now and I suppose that he did save my life. I am always like that, cagey with people I have just met, and even more so with doctors whom I do not know. Funny really, as he saved my life and yet I barely knew him. Plus, I was slightly too drugged up to make any sense of this anyway. I was deeply embedded in a drug cloud, engulfed in a thick fog that seems as if it would never lift. Funny I had not thought of cancer once! So I got straight in to see Mr. Rice, the nurses removed the dressings and the pump so he could have a look, and then the nurses cleaned and redressed the wound. He basically talked to my mother as she was the main carer and told her what instructions to pass onto the district nurse, and he then asked me to come see him again next week.

The next three weeks flew by in a blur. I was still very much out of it and still very much in pain. The vac pump was wearing us all down as it was still giving problems. My next visit to Mr. Rice was not such a positive one. When the nurses took down the dressing and removed the pump, he had a look and was not happy. He told me he was going to have to keep me in if there was a bed available, because the wound needed to be cleaned out surgically and the pump was not working at all. He then said that he was going to try and place some skin grafts on the wound. There were some points on the wound where it was not that deep and that's where he wanted to try placing the grafts. He was going to take some skin from my thigh and place it on the wound and hope that it would take. Fingers crossed that it would work. Not another stay in hospital! I know he said to expect them but really, did I have to? All I wanted to do was to go home and pretend this whole nightmare had never happened.

We had to wait to find out whether there was a bed available and I was secretly hoping there would not be. But of course there was and my mother had to go home to get some of my stuff together. Here I was, stuck on a hospital bed wishing my life away. I was jealous of everyone around me that was not a patient, jealous that they could walk out of here anytime they felt like it, jealous simply that they could take life for granted. I really missed my life, though I had almost forgotten what that actually felt like. Everyone was a great support really, but my mother was the best of all. Karen was another great person. She had had the dogs for so long; I would have had to rehome those dogs if it was not for her. I was really really lucky to have such fantastic friends and they were all a great support. I was really frustrated and I did not have a clue what lay ahead of me, only that is was going to be a long, scary road.

The next morning came and they wheeled me down to theatre. After a few hours I woke up and the pain was unbearable. I had the usual pain in my leg, as well as the throbbing wound pain. and now I had an extremely uncomfortable pain from where he had removed the skin. Ouch!!!!! I was still so heavily medicated that I slept the evening away. The next morning Mr. Rice came around and he was ever so hopeful that the grafts would work. Fingers and toes

88

crossed. I was slowly starting to get to know and like Mr. Rice. I actually felt looked after and safe. Weird I know, but I guess when somebody is looking after you and saves your life, a type of special connection is formed. That's what it felt like anyway.

A couple of days later I could still barely get out of bed, not to mind bear cleaning the wounds and having my dressings changed. Mr. Rice decided to let me go home. He mentioned that if the skin grafts worked, he might have to do some more of them, and if they did not, I might have to come in and get the wound cleaned out surgically again, and then he might try exposing it to the air for a few hours a day. Because I lived near the sea, the salty air would do wonders for it. So now I had a rough idea of what he was planning for me for the next few weeks, and yet I was not sure what route I wanted to take at all. All I knew was that I was in extreme pain.

The journey ride home was absolutely agony. I could barely walk as it was and now I had this problem. The wounds, where he had removed the skin, felt like carpet burns magnified a thousand times. It was so painful. It took me what seemed like an eternity to get out of the car into the wheelchair and into the house. I went straight to bed. I was still in major agony and I had to look forward to the district nurse coming the following day to do the bandage change.

The next morning came and I awoke to the arrival of the district nurses. In hindsight, it was good that two of them had come because this was not going to be pleasant for any of us. Normally I am very quiet and I never, or try not to, complain too much when they are doing the bandage change. The worst part is always removing the dressing, the rest is normally quite bearable. But on this day, from the minute they started, the pain was so excruciating that I roared the house down, begging them to stop. One of the nurses had to tell my mother to leave the house because she knew how hard my family found it to witness such an event. My reaction, while it may have seemed over the top, was very much warranted, because the pain was nothing like I ever experienced in this world, and I will never forget it either. I found myself hating Mr. Rice at that moment in time for the mere suggestion of skin grafts.

When they finished there was a collective sigh of relief, none greater than my own. We then discussed the next bandage change and they planned to get some kind of painkiller for me to take an hour prior to having the dressing changed. I was glued to the bed and did not move away from it. Mom was still trying to give me some food through the peg feed but it kept making me feel sick, and it was not long before we gave up on it. My appetite was slowly starting to return, though I was still not able to eat a great deal. I slept for most of that day, the pain having exhausted me.

The next week flew by and, though still extremely painful, I was managing to tolerate the bandage changes better than that fateful first time. When it came to seeing Mr. Rice that day, the nurse said to organise an ambulance, as I still found it way too hard and too painful to move. So the ambulance arrived and took us in to see Mr. Rice and it felt weird to be stretchered in to see him. I decided I liked him again, but I still have not forgiven him for the grafts. I might though if they worked!! So again, the nurses took down the dressing and Mr. Rice came in and took a look. It was still too early to tell, but he said some of it had taken and that we would give it until next week to know for sure. But other than that he was happy with my progress. I was starting to become more aware of my surroundings. Finally, small clearings were appearing in the fog.

I got the ambulance home, and I did my usual stint of lying in bed watching a bit of TV and having a nap. I still was not able to get out of bed and actually walk. The skin grafts had really set me back. The week just drifted by and before I knew it they had the ambulance outside the door again for me.

When I got to see Mr. Rice, I learned that all our

efforts had been to no avail, as the grafts had failed to bind to the host area. Great, back to the drawing board, though this guy was obviously not giving up. He then said what I hated to hear. He wanted me to stay in again, just for a few days, so the wound could be cleaned out and then exposed to the air for a few hours a day. I admired his gutsy approach. In fact I could now see that he was far from being a typical consultant. He treated me like a human being, not like a piece of meat as some surgeons did. I was still dependent on the wheelchair, as I found it really hard to walk. My energy levels barely hovered above zero. I had, however, stopped using the gastric tube. So, minor little achievements for me. The looming hurdle now was this wound. I finally managed to persuade one of the nurses to take a photo of it and My God! It was as if a grenade had been set off between my buttock cheeks. I was wondering where the hell my anus was? The size of the wound was the biggest I have ever seen, completing dwarfing my tumour removal wound.

So here I was again, once more stuck in hospital in the Clonfert Ward. Kerry General was becoming my second home. It wasn't the worst of second homes I guess, but I was beginning to miss my dogs terribly. The next day I was brought up to theatre, and I realised that I had seen all these theatre nurses more than my friends over the last couple of months. I was worried in case I was going to turn into one of those people that became addicted to surgeries!! I liked the part where they put you to sleep, but that was all. After a few hours, I awoke once more and waited for my usual tea and toast. I was really becoming an old hand at this.

The next day came, and Mr. Rice came in from his rounds that morning and said that today the wound was to be exposed for a good few hours, so I would not be going anywhere. I thought he was out to torture me in some way or punishing me for ruining his Christmas or something!!! So I had to lie down on my stomach and the nurse came in and removed the dressing. She then cleaned the wound and covered it lightly, whilst still leaving it exposed to the air. Boredom was now another hurdle to combat. I tried sleeping for a while, yet time seemed to stumble on as slowly as I could ever remember.

On the day he allowed me home, he told me that the district nurses would call every day and that I was to have the wound exposed for two hours a day. It was not as if I had anything better to do anyway! He also said that he wanted me to get out of the wheelchair, once we got a handle on the wound. The thought of this did not particularly cheer me, as I could not walk all that much due to the loss of muscle mass.

The next week flew by, and the day before I went in to see Mr. Rice, a physio called to the house. The whole experience left me both upset and depressed. I found that when I tried getting out of bed I could not place my left foot fully flat on the floor. The muscles in the back of my calf had fully tightened up and I basically could only walk in a tip-toe fashion. The physio said that I would need a Botox injection in the back of my foot and that freaked me out all together. She then said that I would never be able to walk without the aid of crutches, which seriously depressed me.

The next day, when I went in to see Mr. Rice, I told him what had transpired with the physio which he dismissed, saying that I did not need an injection. He also said that we would try to loosen out that muscle by using a cast and that it would be less painful for me. I was relieved. He examined my wound and was really pleased with what he saw. It was far from being healed but was looking really well. So I went out to the plaster room and the man stretched out my leg as much as he could and plastered it to just below the knee. It was uncomfortable for a while. I was not to see Mr. Rice for another two weeks, so things were really looking up. It was funny what was becoming normal in life, this routine of hospital and home had now become my reality.

So I started getting out of bed more often. I started using the Zimmer frame for a while and then progressed to the crutches. I was nearly out of breath by the time I got to the sitting room! I only managed to stay up for an hour but it was another small achievement. Energy levels were still negligible, though very slowly improving. Some days seemed to drag, others were not so slow. I still had the catheter, gastric tube and the colostomy in place. The colostomy was a necessary evil, something that I resented while at the same time realising that defecating like a normal person would have been a nightmare for me. I knew it was only temporary and there was nothing wrong with it. It did, however, take a long time to get used to the bags, making sure they were stuck on securely. I was paranoid about it, self-conscious to the extreme, but I knew that it was vital. I know that there is a stigma to colostomies and a number of misconceptions. I just want to make clear that the bags do not stink unless they are not secured properly. I further consoled myself with the thought that my anus was a lot cleaner than most other people's!!!

Two more weeks left to go with the cast. My nephew's Holy Communion was fast approaching. My mother and Aunt Cecilia took me to Tralee to buy an outfit for the occasion. I felt that I would not be up for much on the day, but I would go over for an hour or two nevertheless, as the party was being held at their home. I was getting around using a mixture of crutches and the wheelchair because I tired very easily. I was still on very strong painkillers and tablets for my nerves. Shane, Liz, Patrick and baby Joseph were due home soon also. So we were all excited to see them. All we had seen of Joseph was through Skype. He looked like a very handsome baby and I was looking forward to meeting him for the first time.

I was now gradually staying up for longer periods of time, no more than two hours, but still another little achievement. The week flew by. The nurses were very happy with the healing process, though my wound was still very large. Mr. Rice was also happy with the progress I was making and felt that the time was approaching to have the catheter removed. He also tried to remove the gastric tube but to no avail. So he said he would refer me to a Mr. Murray. It was nearly going on May already. It felt like time was going so slow for me and yet the months were flying by.

I got the call to see Mr. Murray for the next day, so it was all go. I was a bit nervous meeting a new doctor. By this stage, I had experienced the whole gamut of medical staff in Kerry General and to every man and woman they were absolutely fantastic. The hospital impressed me immensely. Everyone was so supportive and caring. The next day arrived and I was immediately brought into a room to wait for Mr. Murray. I wondered what he was like. Generally I let Peggy do all the talking but I would wait and see. When he came in the door he instantly put me at ease and he seemed a very down-to-earth kind of guy. He told me he had heard all about me and my case. He also had heard that I was a dog lover, adding that he had two himself, of whom he showed me pictures. He even asked if I had pictures of my own dogs. I instantly liked him very much. We discussed the options of removing the gastric tube and he agreed to do it under full anaesthetic, because I was a little too afraid to brave it under local anaesthetic. I felt so comforted and assured by the staff of Kerry General that I never wanted to be treated anywhere else. Any remaining treatment I had to undergo I wanted to do so here.

The procedure was scheduled for two weeks time, and next week was the Holy Communion. At home, the boredom was sometimes a killer and I think I was now smoking more then I had ever done. I knew I needed to come off them and considering I hadn't finished the cycles of chemotherapy, I should have been careful.

Shane, Liz and the kids arrived, and it was lovely to see them. I spent most of my time between the living room and bedroom. I tried to stay up as long as I could, but I tired easily. They were understanding though, and they came down to the bedroom to me rather than me having to go up to be with them. Patrick was a lively fellow but very sweet, and Joseph was the spitting image of Shane - quite a gorgeous little fellow. I could barely hold him in bed, but somehow I managed. I had always loved babies and I could not go without holding him and spending as much time with him as possible.

My nephew Ronan's Communion day arrived quickly. This was the first significant social occasion I had to face since my brush with death. I was only going to the house, as what energy I had, I wanted to spare for the party. I was conscious of all the tubes hanging out of me, though I think I managed to cover them all up successfully. I hoped so anyway. When we arrived there were a lot of people there, and I feared that it was not going to go well, as my attention span was not that great. I hadn't seen some of these people in ages. Was I going to be able for it? Though, admittedly, it was a little late for doubts now.

So I plastered a smile on my face and slowly got out of the car. Aidan had organised a wooden ramp for the wheelchair to get into the house and there was a marquee outside as well. So I plonked myself next to Jane, Katie's sister, and near her boyfriend Ger. I thought it would be easier to begin with, being outside in the marquee. So I ate a bit of food and talked to Jane for a while. Then I got wheeled into the house and I had no choice now but to talk to a few people. I meant no offence to them but I was in no fit state to be there really, as my attention span was non-existent and I could not concentrate on any of the conversations around me. I was enjoying it, but trying to take part in conversations was extremely tiresome.

After an hour or so, I said to Shane that I had no choice but to go home because I was going to drop otherwise. It was the longest time I had been out of the bed, not to mention the longest time in another house, other than Kerry General!!! I said my goodbyes to everyone, and Ronan looked happy, so that was the main thing. Shane and Liz were now talking about having Joseph's christening at my house. Considering how long I had been up for I thought, 'Oh crap, where's that energy going to come from!!!!' But I was getting stronger by the week and they were talking about having it in August, so hopefully I would have recovered much more energy by then. I was also honoured, because they asked me to be Joseph's Godmother. So that would be something to look forward to and motivate me to set a goal to become more mobile and to have more energy. There was a lot to organise for it and I said I could help out, even if it was just from bed. What little I could do, I would do.

The rest of that weekend went fast and Shane and Liz went back to Paris on Monday. I was also due in Kerry General to have my gastric tube removed which, thankfully, was just a day procedure. I realised that it was now May, and so it had been six months since my encounter with the big scary abscess. I have come a long way since then. So I was admitted and had a bit of a wait, but eventually I got down to theatre and it was over before I knew it. When I got back to the day ward, one of the nurses said that once I had my tea and toast, she would organise someone to come up and remove the cast, and that Mr. Rice would be up to see me before I went home. After an hour, a man came up and removed the cast. It felt good to have the cast removed and to be one tube less. Mr. Rice arrived and he checked my walking with the crutches, without the cast, asking me if I had noticed an improvement since last time. I said that it was much better as I could now walk more on the flat of my foot. He then said he would organise physio and he asked me where would suit better, Listowel or Tralee? I said Tralee immediately, remembering the last time I was there. He also said to start walking on the sand at the beach.

The wound was doing extremely well and it was being exposed to the air every two hours. It was actually getting smaller. One night, however, I woke in terrible pain gripped by the sensation that I needed to go for a pee and yet not being able to. We had to call South Doc. After an hour or two, a doctor arrived and he informed me that the catheter was blocked. The minute he released the air bubble from the catheter, I cried with the relief of release. I apologised as I could not stop the urine from coming. What dignity I once had was now well and truly by the wayside. He then had to insert a new catheter. I hated the feeling of them going in. Why is it always at night these things happen to me? It's bloody typical. The night after that, I had to call South Doc again, as the catheter had come undone, and when the doctor eventually arrived I asked him if it would not be better just to leave it out, as Mr. Rice wanted it gone soon anyway. But the doctor said no and put another one in. I was really getting fed up of it.

Another day during the weekend, they had to call a further two times and they kept inserting a new one each time. It was really starting to irritate me. On Monday, the day that President Obama came to Moneygall, I was lying in bed when I felt something pop. I put my hand down to feel what had happened and there was the catheter having come out by itself, inflated and all. Luckily, this time it occurred during the working hours of my usual GP, Dr. O'Reilly, I told him what had occurred over the weekend, so he decided in the end that it was better not to bother putting it back in. I think my body was starting to

101

reject it anyway. I had the commode, so my mother placed that by the bed because it was going to take a while before my pelvic floor muscles would start working properly, even though I was doing the exercises in preparation for the catheter being removed. So another little achievement. I was nervous and yet at the same time happy, knowing that I was making improvements no matter how slow it felt.

It was now the end of May and another two months to the christening. I had to go in to see Mr. Rice again and he was thrilled that the catheter was finally out and that I had organised a physio appointment for the next day. He was also happy with the wound, as it had decreased dramatically in size, so things were really looking up. He gave out to me though, because he felt that I was using the wheelchair too much. I therefore committed myself to walking more.

I was now sitting up in the sitting room for much longer. My energy levels were increasing to a certain extent. I couldn't believe how long it was taking to recover to what I remembered being a normal state of health. I was still very far off, but I was slowly getting there. I loved how it is portrayed in films, that when the good guy gets shot or seriously sick and spends the obligatory couple of weeks or months in the ICU, they seem to thereafter make this miraculous recovery and are suddenly back to work within a day or two of leaving hospital. To Hollywood screenwriters, it does not work that way at all. It's far from it!!!

The next day came and I went in for physio to find out that I had Finn, who had worked with me in my ICU days. It was good to have someone I knew and he knew me. He was a real taskmaster and worked me hard for the hour. My leg hurt like hell but it was worth it because it all helped my leg to recuperate strength and mobility. He said I had lost a lot of muscle over my buttocks and that I would need a high protein diet to help regain the muscle that I had lost. He could not answer my tough questions, like whether I would ever be able to walk without the help of a crutch or a cane. But he did not say no, like the others had in the past. I was grateful to him as he gave me hope for the future, hope that I might one day get back to work.

When I got home I was stiff as a poker. The next few weeks were physio and more physio, and indeed my leg was getting gradually stronger. I was starting to use the wheelchair less often. It was limited now to only when it rained, because I was afraid of slipping and Mom was a bit nervous of me when I went out as well. I also started to cook again, nothing elaborate, for I could not do a whole lot. Again, my mother had to help me because I could not stand over the hob for very long. I was finding it very hard to stand for long periods and also sitting down on most chairs was a literal pain in the bum. I brought it up with Finn on my next session with him and he said this discomfort was due to the lack of muscle in that area. Basically, when I was standing and leaning on my bad leg, all that was supporting that leg upright was pure bone, save for a very small amount of muscle, and again when sitting down I was sitting on my prosthesis, with no muscle or extra padding. So therefore, I had a lot of work to do in order to acquire enough muscle for me to be able to stand for longer than two minutes and also for me to be able to sit.

It was now the middle of June and my wound was almost completely healed. Mr. Rice was very pleased that I managed to walk into his consulting room with the aid of crutches. He was also delighted with the healing process. He said that it wouldn't be long now before the wound could be closed and that I could then have the colostomy reversed. He seemed dead pleased with himself, and so he should. My admiration for him had grown incrementally throughout my recovery and, indeed, if I had to undergo any further treatment, I would have loved to have him involved. I knew he was not an oncologist, but I trusted his judgment. I hoped he was willing because I had yet to ask him. I also decided if I was obliged to have anymore chemotherapy treatment that it was going to be down in Tralee. Even if Professor Carney said no! I had not heard anything from Professor Carney since the abscess incident, and Mr. Rice has mentioned nothing about chemotherapy or him, so I guessed there was no point in worrying about it for another few months anyway.

In the middle of July, Finn managed to get me walking with the use of canes. It was much more strenuous as it called upon a lot more muscles and I walked a hell of a lot straighter. He said to only use them at home for now, until I got stronger using them. I was euphoric. By this time, the wound was more or less healed, though it still had to be cleaned and I still had to be careful because the scar tissue was still very tender. Mr. Rice and the district nurses were really pleased with the outcome, as it had taken a long seven or eight months to get it to heal fully. So another milestone was achieved.

The christening was coming ever so fast. After a week, the stoma (colostomy) started to prolapse, which means a bit of the intestine had started to bulge out. I organised to meet the stoma nurse and she explained that it had probably happened because I was getting more active, and also due to the use of the more strenuous canes. So she advised me not to use the canes for a while, until the stoma was reversed. I had

105

to see Mr. Rice and he said not to get the stoma reversed for a while, because the wound has just healed and it needed a couple of weeks to strengthen up. Great, I had to go around the place with this big lumpy thing on my belly. But I managed to conceal it the best way I could and it actually worked. That was the only trouble I ever got from the stoma, so I could not really complain.

I kept practicing staying up longer for the christening, so that I would be able to enjoy it without feeling too exhausted. I also tried to go back driving again and it was such a wonderful feeling. Small drives progressed to longer drives. I was recovering more and more of my independence. Another major achievement. I planned to make a stir fry for the christening, like I did for Ronan's Holy Communion. I was actually looking forward to it. The dogs were also back full-time now and it was great. I spent some time outside playing ball with them and cuddled with them in the sitting room. My little family was back to being half a working unit at least.

August arrived and with it Shane, Liz and the kids. There was a lively buzz to the house and they were delighted to see me being up and about, because the last time they saw me I was stuck in bed with hardly any energy. The hospital bed was now gone and it was great to be back in my own regular bed. On

Wednesday, Aidan, Shane and dad were busy outside putting the marquee up, while the vet came to give the dogs their vaccinations. We then went food shopping on Thursday and I went to physio. I was able to use the canes for that hour. I was now driving myself to the hospital and it was encouraging to be dependent on myself for that at least. I had planned to collect Karen on Saturday for the christening party and bring the dogs up to her for the few hours, as there would be too many people around. I was sore and stiff - the usual effects post a physio session. The pain was welcome though, for it meant that my leg was getting stronger though, admittedly, there was still a long journey to go.

So on Saturday morning I prepared the stir fry and then got myself ready and we all went off to the church. It was a lovely service. Then we all made our way down to the house where everything had been prepared. I kept the dogs there for a while, as Liz`s Mom and Dad were also great dog lovers and I thought it would be nice for them all to meet. It was just us family for the dinner part.

So at 3pm, I left with the dogs to go to Kilflynn to collect Karen and drop off the dogs. When I had returned everyone had turned up to the party, there were even some faces that I haven`t seen since my diagnosis and it was lovely to catch up with them. The day went pretty fast and it was a good day in all. I actually broke a personal record by going to bed really late for the first time in nine months!!! I was shattered the next day. I could not believe how quickly the week flew by. The lads went back to Paris on Monday and the house seemed so quiet without them.

I went in to see Mr. Rice on the Wednesday and I told him how annoying the stoma was because of it prolapsing. So he said he would get onto Mr. Murray in the near future to organise the reversal of the stoma. I was relieved and looked forward to feeling like a normal person again. I knew I look disjointed from a back vista given that I had only half an arse, but to be able to do all the normal things again like a normal person would be great. Not that there was anything wrong with the colostomy, after all it was very necessary to have it, considering where the wound was. Mr. Rice warned me that once reversed, I would be having a few accidents, because of the length of time the muscles back there were out of use. I was seized by a new sense of motivation and resolved to diligently practice my pelvic floor exercises.

The next day I had physio and, again, I felt very sore and stiff afterwards. I still had the cancer to worry about, but to tell you the truth, the ordeal of the abscess had completely monopolised my attention. Whether that was a good thing or not, I was not quite that sure. Mr. Rice made light of it the last time I mentioned something to do with the cancer issue. I guess he never saw me as being a cancer patient, and in a way that was refreshing. It gave me hope for the future also. It really did help having a supportive and caring doctor during an ordeal like this. I just wished I had him when I was first diagnosed. He really had restored my faith in doctors.

I also decided that when I was finished with chemotherapy and I had to do those monthly or six monthly scans, I wanted him to do it because if there was any bad news ahead, I wanted to hear it from him. Why? Because I could be myself with him, I knew him and trusted him. He also had a very soothing voice which I think I could remember from the time of being unconscious in the ICU. As so much of that time was spent in my subconscious, I find it very hard to explain this in words. It's funny what you end up thinking of when you are recuperating from something like this.

The next week flew by and I got an appointment to see Mr. Murray for the following week. It was already mid-August. I could not believe how quickly the time was flying by.

The day of Mr. Murray's appointment arrived. I had forgotten how nice he was. He informed me that I would have to stay in hospital for a week because they had to ensure I made a bowel movement before leaving, in order to ensure that all was working correctly. He knew I was not too happy with that prospect and he looked at me and said, 'Yes, I know about your aversion to staying in hospitals!' So if I came in on the Friday and had the surgery, then he might make a special allowance and discharge me on Monday. I would then come back and see him in his outpatients' clinic that Thursday, to make sure the wound was OK and that my bowels were working. I was happy with that plan. What a very considerate surgeon he was. I liked him very much and he had a very good sense of humour.

The surgery was to take place the first week of September. I was not really looking forward to the prospect of staying in hospital. It has been a while now since I was in hospital and had any surgery. A week before the surgery, I went to see Mr. Rice and he said that he had to organise CT scans of my lungs for Professor Carney, and that as soon as they were done I had to go up and see him. That hit me with a jolt. No, the reality of the cancer was coming back! I asked him if I could not stay there with him and pretend this part was not happening?!!!!!!! He told me it would be alright and I told him I did not want any more chemotherapy, and if I did, I wanted it done down here in Kerry General. He understood where I was coming from and supportively dragged my mind off it by saying that I should do everything one step at a time -

first get the scans done, then see Professor Carney, then see from there. He was right of course. I was just petrified really. I wished I could get my hands on a pair of handcuffs and tie myself to his desk, anything to avoid what was coming. So he said he would try and organise the scans while I was in for the reversal. Great. Why does reality always have to come back and bite you in the arse? In this case half an arse!!

I was admitted on Friday morning for surgery. Katie was with me and I decided to go out for a cigarette at around 8.30am, as there was some delay with the bed or something. As I was going back in I bumped into Mr. Rice who passed me with a knowing smile. He said that he would try to organise the scan for Monday and that I should be down in surgery by early afternoon hopefully. He wished me well and I went back up to the ward.

In the afternoon I was wheeled down to theatre. I was in the waiting area of theatre where the nurses were doing their final checks, when Mr. Murray came over and spoke with me for a few minutes. Then Mr. Rice joined us. They were both in good form and we all chatted for a while. I was then wheeled into theatre, where they hooked me up to monitors and managed to get a vein, and before I knew it I was out like a light. When I awoke, I was in recovery and everything, thankfully, had gone well.

Things looking great

I was now back in the Clonfert Ward which felt strangely familiar, especially seeing all the nurses again. Everyone was thrilled to see how well I was doing. I was really so very fond of them all. They were all very good to me when I needed them the most. I had a portable DVD player and a Nintendo to keep myself occupied and I was in and out for a cigarette a couple of times. My insides felt sore due to all the internal poking about to make sure my bowels were working properly. I also met up with the usual security guys, who had also become my friends over time. I only saw them every so often, because it depended on who was on when I was coming in for physio or to see Mr. Rice, but I had formed a bond with them all.

The weekend actually passed really quickly and before I knew it, it was Monday morning and time for Mr. Murray's rounds. I had made no bowel movement and I knew he was probably a little bit uncomfortable about releasing me, but he was a man of his word, bless him. I had to come in again on Thursday. He said I would be sore as he did have to poke around there a fair bit, but the wound was good. He placed a mesh before he closed up, in order to prevent a hernia from occurring. So I thanked him and I got ready to go. As I was on my way home, I realised that I had forgotten to get the scan done. I did not feel rushed to do so, as I wanted to recover from this first anyway, and I really had to mentally prepare myself again for all the cancer crap that lay ahead. I decided I was going to go to Dr. O'Reilly at some stage, to see if I could get some help to quit smoking. I think it was definitely time to give them up.

The physio was off for a while as he was getting married, which suited me as I was recovering from the reversal. So by mid-September, I was fit and able to resume my physical rehabilitation. I was now able to use the canes more and my leg had become much stronger. We managed to get through a lot more work during my hour of physio. I was always sore, stiff and tired after it, but it was all worth it. I was also collecting Karen's girls from school each evening and it was great having something to do, as the boredom sometimes got too much.

Before I knew it, October had arrived, so I contacted Mr. Rice and made an appointment to see him. When I got in to see him, he was delighted to see that I was walking, but this time, unfortunately, I was here to see him because of the subject of cancer.

114

Before the scans I had to get some blood tests done. I also asked him if he could be the one to organise my six-monthly scans once I was finished with the chemotherapy, and also, of course, if he could stay involved with my case. I think he very much intended to do so by his answer, and I was ever so pleased. I know I hero-worshipped the man, but when you are sick it is vital that you have a doctor that you like and respect and trust.

I am not saying I didn't trust Professor Carney, but my relationship with him was very different .I had great respect for him and also liked him a lot. I still did not want to go back up to Dublin though. I told Mr. Rice this and he laughed at me, saying all would be fine and not to worry. Easy for him to say. I wish he could come with me!!!! It's funny what the mind thinks of when you are running scared and not wanting to go back on that lonely road of being a cancer patient again. But on the upscale of things, I now had Mr. Rice, and it was good to know that I had a doctor like that behind me. I left his consulting room and went to get the blood test. After a week or so, I got the appointment for the CT scan. I started to worry now, because I hadn't being scanned in months, and what if something showed up? I tried futilely to keep busy as much as possible.

It was raining on the day of my scan so I used
115

the wheelchair. I made straight for the X-ray department. It took a while to get scanned, but I got there in the end. After waiting around for a while, I decided to venture down to outpatients, hoping that I would not see Mr. Rice because he would probably kill me for being in the wheelchair. When I got down there, all the nurses thought I was going into see him, until I explained I was just waiting for my father to collect me. They didn't seem to listen to me, however, as before I knew it I was being pushed into Mr. Rice's consulting room. He was seated there already and appeared in good form. He looked at me and asked if I had already had my scan done. He then gave out to me for using the wheelchair. Great, I knew I was going to get that from him!! I apologised and told him that I was too afraid of slipping in the rain. He replied that next week when I was coming in to see him, I had better be walking in to see him. He was right really. I had to get over that fear of falling, and I had to get my mother to stop too, because her fretting was definitely not helping me.

I had physio the next day and Finn tried something new, something that I was not expecting to happen so soon. He told me to leave the canes and try walking sideways on my own. I looked at him at first, deciding he had gone mad, as I did not think I was ready. But I did what I was told and I found myself

116

doing it. I could not believe it. I was actually walking on my own even if it was sideways. I walked up and down the room and then he said to walk normally front ways. I was a bit slow and a bit wobbly at first, so I had to hold onto him for a while, but then I got steadier on my feet and, hey presto, another major milestone achieved. One that I had certainly not anticipated happening so soon.

I was so delighted I rang my mother, as she had accompanied me to physio, and told her to come up as she absolutely had to see something. When she came up I walked towards her. She was in shock. I don't think she saw that one coming either. As you can imagine, we were in such great form leaving, that I decided to call over to Aidan and Katie and surprised them by walking on my own. They were naturally delighted for me. I called over to Karen to show her and she was thrilled. Niamh and Margaret called over that evening and I surprised them too. I felt like jumping for joy.

The very next day I went to see Dr. O'Reilly and asked him for help to give up cigarettes. I had heard about this tablet that helped with the cravings called Champix and he duly prescribed me some. There was a long list of side-effects, so I decided to show it to Mr. Rice in order to see whether it was worth taking them or not.

117

The next week arrived suddenly and I was quite anxious to hear these results. I went in on my own and I said to him, 'Before I hear the results, you must see something', and he looked curiously at me and asked, 'What?' I then walked around the room without the stick, very stiffly and gingerly, but I walked nonetheless. He was happy to see me managing it, but did not seem at all that surprised that I would be able to do it. Those initial comments from that physio, saying that I would never be able to walk without the aid of a stick, had obviously affected me so much that I lost faith in myself that way.

I noticed Mr. Rice smiling at this stage and wondered what was so amusing. 'The results are clear, your lungs and liver look good', he said. What an inexpressible huge sigh of relief! He then said that I should make an appointment to see Professor Carney straight away. I looked at him and he probably could see the fear in my eyes. I blurted out something about not wanting chemotherapy. But he simply reassured me, saying that I would be fine, and if I had any problems to get on to him. I also showed him the leaflet showing the list of Champix side-effects, and asked if it would be alright to take them? He had a look and said that he couldn't see any reason that would prevent me from taking them. He was delighted that I was even trying to give them up.

The strangest and most scary thing now was that I was not going to see Mr. Rice until after Christmas, for the next scan. I guess I was so used to seeing all the medical staff here that I found it hard to let go or something. How lucky I had been with both doctors and nurses here. I also guess that I associated them with a treatment distinct from cancer, and now it was time to face up to that reality again.

So I grew a backbone and made an appointment to see Professor Carney. I decided that I was going to go up and see him myself. My Uncle Noel kindly offered to share the driving and Shane was to fly in from Paris to meet us in Dublin. I think I needed to distance myself from my close circle of carers for this. I had not told Shane that I was walking on my own, not that I was doing it constantly though, as my leg was still not strong enough for that yet. I could not wait to see him and his face when he saw me walking on my own.

The day came and we left early, and it felt really strange to be going up to Dublin, as I had not been there since before the abscess. A strong tide of mixed emotions ebbed and flowed inside me. I was really anxious about the thoughts of having more chemotherapy. When we had arrived and parked, I brought my stick and the wheelchair, as it was too far to walk. As we were walking towards the hospital, we

119

saw Shane coming towards us, so I told Noel to stop. I got up from the wheelchair and started to walk towards him. He was thrilled and surprised and said that he would not tell Liz, as they were coming home the following week and I could surprise her as well.

We had arrived far too early, so we went for dinner and then headed down to the waiting area. My nerves were running around in circles like a washing machine in my stomach. I still had time to bolt, except alas, I could not run!!! Professor Carney then called me in. We talked about the abscess for a while, how great Mr. Rice had been and how lucky I was to have had him as my consultant. Then he said the one thing I most wanted him to say, that there was no point in having any more chemotherapy, because it had been a year since I had undergone the 6th cycle of treatment, and the scans were good and long may that last. So all was hopeful and I was now in remission. Fingers, toes and everything else crossed that I would stay that way. I was so relieved and delighted. I gave him a big hug before I left. As I was leaving, he asked me to come and see him again in six months' time after the next scan. The relief...did this mean I could get my life back again and live again?

Shane walked us back to the car and we were all in a very good mood. I rang Mom to tell her the good news. I then rang Mr. Rice's secretary and asked if I could speak to him. She told me that he would ring me back within the hour. So we settled into the journey back home and after a half hour passed, Mr. Rice rang back. I told him the good news and he was delighted. I did not have to see him again until January, which was the time for my next scan. I felt great, I felt like shouting it from the tallest building around. No more hospitals, no more scans! Well, for a little while at least. I was going to be exhausted when I got home and I had to go to physio the next day, but the celebrations at home took precedence over everything.

The next day, when I got in to see Finn, I had some more good news, as he told me that he envisioned me getting back to work in around three months' time. Whoopee. So I started taking the Champix tablets immediately. The idea was that I was to carry on smoking until day 11, whereupon then I was then to stop and go cold turkey. I began the treatment without any discernible side-effects over the first few days. Things really seemed to be progressing. My mother had, at this stage, moved back to her own house and I was now doing a lot of basic things for myself.

Finn suggested that I take up swimming, as this would be the best exercise for my leg and assist in regaining some muscle. This required some research, as I could not go into a normal swimming pool, as there had to be steps into the pool. Finding one was not going to be easy. I was kept really busy now because I had to do things for myself for a change. By the end of the evening, my lower back and the bad side of my hip ached. But I guess it was a good sign because I was obviously using muscles I had not used in months, which were in sore need of use. If I was going to go back to work, I needed to be able to do a lot more. So I started to go for walks down the road near my house, unfortunately though without my dogs, as my leg was still not strong enough for that yet.

The following week, I drove down to Cork to collect Shane and his family once more. I could not believe it was the end of October already. Some people were quick to remind me that Christmas was coming, and it would be a year since the abscess. I found that I did not like being reminded of this, as it made me feel very uncomfortable and I was not looking forward to Christmas at all. I did not think Christmas would ever be the same for me again. Perhaps a little dramatic, but that was the way I was feeling right now. God knows what way I would feel when December came knocking on the door.

I had been off cigarettes three days at this stage thanks to the Champix, and so far so good. I had my moments though, and the evenings in particular were the worst. It was now Halloween and I found welcome distraction in seeing all the kids dressed up and going out trick or treating.

Next thing I knew, it was November. My bowels were still bothering me. I had a nagging, uncomfortable pain as a constant companion and found that I could not go anywhere in the mornings as I was endlessly in and out of the toilet. I hadn't had any accident so far, but I had come close once or twice. By mid-November the problem was still persisting, and I was becoming tormented, as I could not go anywhere or form a routine of any sort. So when I went in for physio that week, I mentioned it to Finn, who advised me that I should make an appointment with Mr. Murray, just to make sure. So I did. I did not want any lingering issues like this in January when I went back to work.

I made the appointment to see him for the following week. I was grateful to Finn, as otherwise I probably would never have thought of contacting Mr. Murray. Meanwhile, I had found a swimming pool, but I only managed to go a few times as my bowels got the better of me and I was too afraid of an accident happening. God, imagine in the pool! Not even worth thinking about! I depended from time to time now on Imodium tablets which helped me to become more mobile - but only as a last resort.

The following week, I went so see Mr. Murray,

explaining the situation with my bowels, and he suggested I see a physiotherapist who deals specifically with pelvic floor muscles. He also advised me in relation to diet. So I was to try that for a couple of weeks and to come back to him and let him know if this had lead to any improvement. I was willing to try anything. I had two weekly physio appointments, fortunately on different days. I went to see the pelvic floor physio the following week, who wanted to consult with Mr. Murray to see what muscle mass remained. She gave me instructions on the types of exercise to do and how often a day they should be repeated. These were going to keep me more than busy for the next month or so, following which, there would hopefully be signs of improvements.

Another milestone when I decided to ring Mr. Rice to see whether it was possible to get the port channel removed, as it was not working and I was finished treatment. He said he would say it to Mr. Murray and try to arrange an appointment for me. So after a week or two, I got an appointment to see Mr. Murray the following Thursday morning. I was a bit nervous as I had quite a break from all the needles, etc. Thursday morning came, and I went in and met all the nurses in outpatients where we had a good catch up. I was then called in to one of the procedure rooms. I had to put on a gown just in case my clothes would get destroyed.

Mr. Murray came in and instantly put me at ease, and asked me if I wanted to be sedated or if I would just prefer to have the local anaesthetic. I decided I was going to be totally positive and consider this to be my last surgical treatment, so I said I would be brave and go for the local anaesthetic. I was nervous, but again Mr. Murray and all the nurses put me at my ease. The sensation was weird and he had to tug at the port channel a little to get it out. He did a lovely job at sewing me up - that scar was going to look a lot better than the one that was there from when it was put in in Dublin. So I got through it and I was feeling very proud of myself. I don't think I would have gone through it only for Mr. Murray and the nurses being such a great support to me once again.

And then December came. Memories, what do you do with them especially ones that you were not sure you even wanted? I decided I was going to leave most things to the last minute. This December, I was not going to take anything for granted. I still had people come up to me and say 'My God, it's been a long year for you!' I felt like telling them to shut up. I really just wanted to try and forget the whole thing. But I knew they meant well so I smiled and agreed with them.

On the 15th of December, the anniversary of the

abscess incident, I had one or two people ring me, to express solidarity I guess. Being reminded of it tormented me and I began to find that I really did not like Christmas anymore. My bowels had good days and bad, but overall I did not notice any discernible improvement. I was in contact with work and organised to return towards the end of January - So plenty of time. I was nervous with the thoughts of meeting everyone again, but at the same time I was eager to get back.

So Christmas was here and the family was all around, and yet my head was awash with feelings that I could not control. Keeping busy helped. The only thing I enjoyed about Christmas now was Andrea Bocelli's Christmas songs. Apart from that it felt like any other normal day of the week. On Christmas Eve though, the tree looked beautiful, full of presents underneath it ready to be opened, and I did begin to feel a little festive. Aidan's family arrived to join in our usual exchange of gifts. It was really nice to have everyone around. They made a speech to mark the occasion saying how glad they were that I was here to share it with them, mindful of last year. I got the best present ever that I began to count down the months to immediately - Andrea Bocelli concert tickets for November 2012! The best present I have ever gotten and I was already excited. All the children seemed

126

equally happy with their presents. What remained of Christmas passed uneventfully, and it was indeed nice, but I was glad it was over. I seem to have irrevocably lost the Christmas spirit.

It was ever so close to going back to work now and I was starting to get quite nervous. Though to begin with, I was only to do a few hours and start very slowly. Before I knew it the day arrived, and there I was getting up early to get ready and making sure that I had gone to the toilet before I left. I was making my way to work and just before I got to Kilcornan, I had an uncontrollable urge to go to the toilet. Typically, there was no toilet in sight so I had to drive to a service station in the next town. I managed to get there and grab the key, but unfortunately not soon enough to prevent an accident.

This is a very embarrassing subject. I felt extremely low and at a loss to understand why one day it went one step forward, only for the next day to take two steps back. I was now worried that I would not make the rest of the journey, not to mention last the few hours at work. Would I have to return home before I arrived? If an accident happened, how could I face these people? It's not as if I could discuss this problem freely with them. Why was this happening to me now? I took an Imodium and hoped to God that it would work. When I got down there, I was extremely nervous. It was strange and nice being back, and it helped to take my mind off my bowel problems which, typically, had settled down by now anyway.

Those initial hours back at work flew by, and before I knew it, I was on the journey home. Naturally, my bowels did not cause any trouble at all. When I got home, I was really proud of myself considering what had happened that morning, but I was also knackered. I was not due back at work until Saturday and I was already looking forward to it. I was getting my life back ever so slowly. On Friday, I made an appointment with Dr. O'Reilly, in the hope that he could prescribe something stronger then Imodium, in order to help me make the journey without an incident. Perhaps nerves caused it to behave that way? Hopefully, it was nothing more than that.

So on Saturday, I got to Foynes and again I had to make a dash to the toilet, though not before succumbing to another bloody accident. Why was this happening? Why now when I was just getting back to work? A sense of rebellion rose within me, and I took an Imodium to make sure it would not happen again. I managed to make it as far as Kildimo, before having to make another dash, but this time the accident was much bigger. Why oh why? I had never felt so frustrated in my life. I did not know whether to give up and turn around, or take a chance and keep going?

I decided I would keep going and if it happened again, then I would turn around. At least I had an appointment to see Mr. Murray the Thursday coming. This time I got to Patrickswell, before having to make another dash. That's it, I had no choice but to turn around. So I rang work to explain that I could not make it in. I turned around and headed for home. I was never so down in myself. I cried all the way home.

That Thursday, I made it half-way to Tralee, when I had to turn back and get home to go to the toilet. Great, now I couldn't even get to Tralee without an incident. I left to go to Tralee again, and I just made it into Kerry General when I had another accident. Luckily it was happening near a toilet, otherwise I would have been majorly embarrassed.

When I eventually got to see Mr. Murray, I let him have it. Frustration poured out of me, everything that had happened, how desperate I was to have this situation resolved as fast as possible. He could not have been more understanding. He felt that there was a definite weakness in that area and wanted to consult with Professor Masterson and Mr. Rice to find out how much muscle was lost and removed. But it was looking as if I would need surgery. There were, however, several options I could try, before it became so serious that I had no other option but to have the colostomy back again. I did not really fancy that. He advised me

129

not to return to work until this issue was sorted out. I left his room, depressed with the thought that I was, for now, going to be more or less house-bound. When I got home, I had a letter informing me of an appointment to see Mr. Rice, which actually cheered me up in a way, as I had not seen him in ages.

Too Good to be True

The following week, I went in to see Mr. Rice, who was aware that I had only made it into work for one day. He looked as depressed as I was, especially as he had wanted me to go back to work since before Christmas. I'm not sure if in some way he blamed himself, as he apologised to me for having to remove half my anal sphincter, as well as some muscle around the pelvic floor area during a debridement, following my abscess episode. I looked at him incredulously, thinking he had gone mad, for this was no one's fault. He did what he had to do to save my life. Unfortunately, there had to be some collateral damage. I could not get away that lightly. Nobody, however, had anything to apologise for.

It was time for those scans again. He sent me off to have the usual blood test done. As a precautionary measure this time, I was also to have my bowels scanned, in order to ensure there was nothing wrong with them internally. I found it hard now to go anywhere, because it was impossible to judge the behaviour of my bowels, each day was different from the next. But being determined not to let it beat me, I did manage to get it under some sort of control. I was getting out of the house at least. I already had to call a halt to swimming, so I was damn well not going to let it interfere with anything else. Impossible to believe, but it was now the month of February. How time was flying, as it was way back in October when I had my last scan. The following week, I went in to have my scan done, and I was indeed anxious, but more so about my bowels then my lungs, which I guess wasn't any harm, as it took my mind off worrying about cancer too much.

During the week that I waited for the results of the scans, I managed to get out for some walks, which proved to be a good way of clearing my head. How would one ever get used to this business of endlessly waiting for results? The week dragged, and was made even worse, when I was asked a few times whether or not I had got the results back. I kept myself busy as much as possible. By the end of the week, I got a call for an appointment to see Mr. Rice. So what were these results to be, good or bad? What about my bowels? A week of sleepless nights hadn't helped my morale. But I didn't feel as if there is anything wrong me, apart from my malfunctioning bowels, so hopefully all was good.

I helped Karen out this week by collecting the girls for her, anything to distract my mind from what was coming. How could I keep doing this every six months? It was no way to live, having to contend with this constant nagging worry. The fear of it coming back was never far from my mind - especially after what had happened last year. But I had to put it out of my mind, and hope for the best and for the future. I was really more worried now about my bowels, because Mr. Rice had mentioned that I may need to have the colostomy back again, and I was really hoping that would not be the case.

So after a sleepless night, it was time to go in and see him. It felt like any other normal visit. Though when I arrived, and took one look at him, I knew something was up. He looked sad and very down and he said that he had some news for me, news that was not good. Oh God, the bloody cancer was back! He said there were a few spots on my lungs, which seemed to indicate a reoccurrence of the cancer. The bowels were going to be put to the side for the moment.

The fear was back. I had forgotten what it was like. Could this really be happening again? I did not deserve this, especially after the year I had just had. What was the point in it? The one thing that went through my head, was that I was glad to be hearing it from him. Funny really, what goes through your mind. We talked for a while, but he was not his usual chirpy self. Then this awful feeling came over me that I had let him down, after all he had done for me in saving my life. I couldn't believe this was happening again. I had absolutely no symptoms and I felt 100 per cent. He instructed me to collect both past and present scans together, and to make an appointment to see Professor Carney straight away. I was in a state of shock and disbelief, and I think he was too, to a certain extent. We talked some more and he even offered to talk to my mother. I thanked him, but refused, as I was not sure whether I was ready for that just yet.

So the cancer was back. I knew it was. What else could it be, and Mr. Rice was certain as well. So when I got home, I decided to tell Peggy, and made her promise not to tell anyone just yet. I then organised getting the scans from the hospital, rang Professor Carney and made an appointment with him for two weeks' time. The waiting game was going to be unbearable, but I should be used to it by now, I guess. God, I could not believe this was happening to me, what if this was the end? Oh God, what about the dogs? I did not want to die.

I drove up to Karen that night and told her, because it was not something you could say over the phone. I was still in a state of disbelief. I couldn't understand how life could throw this at me? What did I do to deserve this? How was I going to get over it? I was awash with questions, the answers to which floated around on the wind. I told Aidan and Katie next, who were both understandably shocked, and then I told Niamh. I couldn't face telling anyone else for now.

During this time, I tried to occupy myself as much as I could. Anything to silence the searing noise of the wait. Niamh agreed to accompany me to Dublin, and I didn't really wish for anyone else to come along. I wanted to be the one in control of all this. So that morning, I drove us to Limerick, barely arriving in time to catch the connecting train to Dublin. The journey felt endless, but we arrived in the end, and jumped in a taxi to take us to the Mater Private. When we got to the waiting area, we were the only ones there. I was really nervous and I was not sure whether I wanted to hear what he had to say. I tried my best to stay positive. He came out and took the scans, and disappeared for about 10 minutes, after which he then called me in. It was very hard to tell what he was thinking, so I sat and waited. He began by saying that the news was not good.

Basically, there were metastases on both lungs, making it impossible to operate yet, as if he did, it might not remove all the tumours, and therefore he would have to operate again. I would not survive two major operations of this sort. Also, there was no point in having them biopsied because he could tell from the scan that there could be a danger of my lung collapsing. So basically I was fucked. I was really scared.

We agreed that I would have chemotherapy for the next three months, and if by virtue of a miracle it worked and the tumours shrunk in size, then I would get the surgery done. If, however, they stayed the same size or grew I was fucked. My past success record with chemotherapy was not good, so therefore what were my chances now? None I guessed. He also said I could get treated as a day-patient in Kerry General, which made me very happy, and that another oncologist would take over the case. What was the point to life if it was going to throw this shit at you? He was very apologetic and empathetic, but there was nothing left to say really. I was in too much shock, I think. I realised that I was going to die. How was I going to handle this? I was not sure at all.

So, when we got out, we got a taxi and headed back for the train station. I told Niamh just before we sat into the taxi and we were both quiet for a while. I could not believe I was back on this road again, this damned lonely road to nowhereville. One scary road with no end, apart from my own, and that freaked the bejaysus out of me. Dread and panic welled up inside me on the way home. I played cards with Niamh to try and distract myself, and it worked in a way.

When we arrived back to Kerry, I drove Niamh home and I called into Aidan and Katie's. My Mother was also there awaiting my return, and so I broke the news to all of them together. I stayed for as long as I could to talk through the situation, before driving to Kilflynn to tell Karen. I was so shattered by the time I got home that I actually did sleep. I loved the mornings when you just woke up, because just for that one glorious minute of waking, you forgot. Unfortunately it did not last for longer than a minute, as by then memory had also awoken and came crashing towards you, hitting you with the force of a ton of bricks. Dread was the feeling of the day.

Professor Carney mentioned that he would send a letter down to Kerry General to instruct them to prepare for the insertion of a port channel into me. What joy! I hoped at least that it would be Mr. Murray looking after it, as he was the one that removed the last one, and also I knew him. I didn`t think I was going to handle having to deal with a new set of doctors all that well. I was the type of person that could not cope with change very well, and I had been so used to Mr. Rice and Mr. Murray that I had become spoiled. Plus they knew me and my long history.

Shane and Liz were planning to come over in the next three weeks. I hated that I was putting my family all through hell again. I hated this disease, mostly for the way in which it was affecting all my family and friends. I knew I could find acceptance from somewhere, but could they? I hoped so. All I did know was that I needed to once again show a strong front for them, whilst also being realistic so that they were prepared for what was to come.

I received my appointment to have the port channel fitted, by post, and was informed that Mr. McCormack was to be my surgeon. It was all so real now. It was actually happening, this was not a nightmare that I was going to wake up from anytime soon. So the following week came, and Niamh drove me to the hospital to be admitted for 8am. The nurses all knew me and were all extremely sympathetic when they heard my news. At 1.30pm, I was brought down to theatre and Mr. McCormack came over to discuss where he was going to insert the channel. Before I knew it, it was all over. I went back to the day ward, and as was the usual ritual, I waited for tea and toast. A nurse called by to inform me that I needed to go down for an X-ray before going home, to make sure the port was in the right place. So after an hour, I went down and had the X-ray. Thankfully, all was well. I went home and rested.

The next day I informed work, and told everyone else that should know because I did not want them to hear it through the grapevine. I kept busy and on Friday Shane, Liz and the children arrived. My appointment to see the oncologist was for the following Wednesday. Not that I was looking forward to that. On Sunday, my niece's christening took place and it was a lovely reprieve of a day.

By Wednesday, Shane decided that he wanted to come with me to meet the oncologist registrar and the oncologist consultant. When I arrived into the waiting room, the reality once again struck me, and fear, dread and panic all vied for my attention at once. Just then I realised that Mr. Rice outpatients' clinic was today, and at that moment all I felt like doing was running up there and pretending this was not happening. Yes, I was a coward, and yet everyone kept telling me how brave I was. It made me laugh sometimes. Because, someone brave to me, chooses to go into that burning fire to rescue another person. I did not choose to have cancer. I did not have a choice and therefore that did not make me brave. I chose to fight because I wanted to live, my survival instinct had kicked in and besides I had no other choice, unless I wanted to give up and die.

After waiting for a while, I eventually got in to see them. I saw Jeff first and he gave me a rough idea of what treatment they had planned for me. Then the Oncologist came in and they had a closer look at the scans again. They informed me that I would also have to go to Cork to get a bone scan done, and they wanted me to get that straight away. So by the time I got home, I got a call from the hospital, saying they managed to get an appointment for me this coming Saturday at 10.00am. Great, that was the day Shane and Liz were leaving, but I guessed I had no choice in the matter. Something else was taking precedence.

That Saturday morning, I drove half-way down, and my father then took over. I dosed myself up with Imodium, so that my bowels would not play up. We just got into the car park of the hospital when the phone rang, and it was Cork University Hospital saying that a mistake had been made, as the bone scan that I was meant to have done did not actually take place on weekends. I would therefore have to turn around and go back home, and another appointment would be rescheduled next week for me. For pity's sick, I could have spent the last few hours with the lads, rather than enduring a wasted trip down here. So we made our way back home, and the lads waited on for us before they had to leave.

After they left, I had to go and do some food shopping, and as I was doing the shopping, I had another bloody accident. This was the very first time it happened this way, suddenly, without any warning, but luckily I managed to hide my disgust and my discomfort, pay up as fast as possible and rush home to die of embarrassment. I was really at my lowest then. I was so down, I wished I had died on that December when the abscess burst. I wished Mr. Rice had not saved me, so I would not have to be going through this all over again. That was my darker moment, and I have had a few of them now and again, but I pulled myself up and pulled myself together.

On Monday morning, I rang Kerry General to let them know that I did not have the scan after all, and explained what happened. So by Tuesday evening, I got another appointment for Thursday. Once again, my father and I made the three-hour journey down. After a tedious, three-hour wait, I eventually got scanned. The staff were not as nice as the staff in Kerry General. They bluntly told me that I had to get my pelvis and lungs X-rayed, as there were some hotspots. Nobody would explain to me either what the term meant, or what the connotations of the term were. I did not like the treatment there, because no-one seemed willing to explain anything to me, and now I was left with another head full of worry until Wednesday, when I would get the results from the registrar.

Kerry General was so superior to this place. The staff, for one, would never have left me feeling so anxious. I realised they saw a lot of patients, and they were only technicians and nurses, but they lacked any real sense of patient empathy.

The next week dragged and I was constantly worrying over the results of the scan. What if something else showed up? What if it had spread somewhere else? How did I handle that then? Again, a whole load of questions that I was never going to hear an answer to. So Wednesday eventually came, and it was the longest wait ever. I eventually got to see the registrar and he said the scans were pretty OK, just obvious signs of wear and tear. I was never so relieved, because I did not think I could have dealt with more bad news.

He then explained what chemotherapy drugs I was going to be on and the ensuing side-effects. Near the top of list came diarrhoea, and I thought to myself, 'Crap, I am going to have to say something here.' So I explained that I was having some bowel issues that never got resolved because of the diagnosis, and wondered if this would be a major problem. So they organised an appointment to see Mr. Murray straight away. I got the appointment for the following day, and I was to get straight back to them to let them know what course of action Mr. Murray suggested. Great, this could mean another surgery and another hold up, crap.

So the next day loomed. I was kind of glad in a way, because it was a break from talking about cancer and chemotherapy treatments, and I knew Mr. Murray, so that also made it nicer. Strange, that having been diagnosed with cancer for the second time, a disease that was probably going to get the better of me, there I was happy to be talking about bowel issues.

So when he came in and asked me about Cork, I presumed he was referring to the scans, so I replied that all was fine apart from some hotspots. He looked at me strangely, and it now dawned on me that he was referring to my bowel problem, and was not aware that the cancer had shown up again. So I told him what had happened and then went on to explain about the side-effects of the chemotherapy. He advised that the colostomy would probably be best, and after all, I could always have it reversed. He did say though that it was up to me to decide upon the course of action. I hated making decisions, but we discussed it a bit further, and I decided to go ahead with the colostomy. I could not handle the idea of being house-bound, nor running the risk of any kind of infection. So Friday week was to be the op day. I hoped to God I was making the right decision here. I knew Mr. Murray would not do it unless he thought it necessary, and I trusted his judgment a bit more then my own.

Later that week, I went to the cinema to see The

Avengers and enjoyed it immensely. It made me stop and think though, I really loved watching films, and it freaked me out that I may not get to see the next Avengers, if one came out in the next two years. It was really strange sometimes, the way the mind worked. I guessed this was its way of making me face facts, and in the long-term allowing me to cope.

I found that the next week flew, and before I knew it I was once again being admitted for surgery. Mr. Murray knew about my notorious aversion to staying in hospitals, even though it did not really bother me this time because one, I was not smoking and two, I had had a long break from it, so it did not seem all that bad really. By 12.30pm, I was being wheeled down to theatre. When I got in, they had trouble finding a vein, so they had to get one on my ankle, of all places. I absolutely freaked out with that, as it hurt quite a bit. It took a bit longer to drift off. But off to la, la land I went.

When I woke up I had the strangest sense of déjà vu, because I recognised some of the nurses from the ICU. I asked them, quite groggily, if they had been transferred to the recovery ward? One of them laughed, and said no, informing me that I was actually in the ICU. I drifted off to sleep again, and the next time I awoke, there was Mr. Rice looking at me with a very strange look. I was definitely afraid of asking

144

what month it was as this was totally a déjà vu moment. I was starting to worry at this stage, because I was unsure as to why I was in the ICU in the first place. So I asked Mr. Rice if he knew why, and he said that I gave a little bit of trouble, and I was bleeding a little bit from the wound, and Mr. Murray wanted me under observation for the night. Nothing major to worry about thankfully. I gave him a hug with the relief, thankful that it was the same month and day as this morning!!!! It really was the strangest feeling ever.

I slept well that night and the next day I was a little sore, but overall the pain was quite manageable. That morning, Mr. Murray`s Registrar came around and said that since things were quiet, I could stay in the ICU. It was strange seeing all the nurses again, and they all remembered me too. The weekend flew by, and next thing it was Monday morning. Mr. Murray himself came around and said things were good, and I could go home if I wanted to. He was so nice and so accommodating, it was great. So that afternoon, I went home and took it very easy. I was still a bit sore and I guess I would be for the next few days. It was strange having to get used to this all over again; they also suggested that my mother should clean my wound for the next week or so, just to make sure it was healing properly.

Over the next few days, I was healing nicely.

On Thursday, I had an appointment with Mr. Murray, and was also due to meet Denise, the stoma nurse. It was strange to be resting again, as I haven`t had that type of surgery in months. Thursday arrived, and I was starting to feel much better. At the hospital, the nurses were all wonderfully supportive. Mr. Murray arrived and examined me. He felt that the wound was doing well, but he wanted to see it again the following week before signing me back over to oncology. Great, an extra week before I started chemotherapy! I was kind of grateful in a way because I was really dreading that part.

We talked for a while and then Denise came in. She was also pleased with the way it was looking, and we talked through the choices of different bags. The colostomy was not all that bad really, once you managed to adjust to the physical change. Denise was a great support also, which always helped. I obviously would have loved the reversal if they were willing to do it after the chemotherapy, but it was not the end of the world either. It did take an awful length of time to adjust, but hopefully I would get there. It felt good to have my confidence back again, simply to be able to go out and not worry about being too far away from a toilet, or having an accident. That's what made it worth it in the end. I went home happy in a way. I did not have to go back in until the following Friday, and from there it was back to oncology.

Again, as always, I kept myself busy for the rest of the week, and when it came to the time to see Mr. Murray, he was more than happy with the progress I had made, so now he felt confident enough to sign me over to oncology. I was back to being a cancer patient. I thanked him and we talked for a while, and I left saying that I hoped to see him again soon. The following Wednesday, I started chemotherapy treatment once again.

A note from Nurse Denise Thornton

It is certainly my pleasure and privilege to meet and deal with such an honest, selfless and determined young woman.

To have a colostomy was the last thing that Ciara had ever envisaged. The fear regarding the management of a stoma and change in body image were some issues Ciara had to deal with. These issues are all relevant and I would encourage every patient to speak to their nurse specialist regarding them. Our aim as a professional body is to provide an environment that patients can communicate with us in a confidential manner. Share the problems you feel you may have.

Of course Ciara took the challenge, and the

fascinating thing was that every question Ciara asked she was sure she was only 'annoying' me by asking, but these were extremely relevant questions and as I always say there is never a 'silly' question. We also as practitioners can learn from ones questions!

This is a vulnerable time for any patient and it is imperative that time is spent discussing the issues that surround life for a person who now has a stoma, for example appropriate appliances, diet, sport, exercise, relationships and identifying support groups to name but a few. My aim is to support and encourage all these questions so as to try and eliminate fears that one may have. Just because one goes home with a stoma and can change their bag independently and with confidence it doesn't mean that the relationship is complete with your nurse. Don't leave something that you may not be sure about go on for too long. Pick up the phone and make contact with your nurse. This is one of the many things I really appreciate from Ciara.

The mountains that Ciara has had to climb and the way that she has dealt with each mile stone with such ferocity has been an inspiration to my colleagues and I, as well as other patients who have had the pleasure to be in Ciaras company. Thankfully Ciara obliged to come to a group meeting one evening (to be honest I twisted her arm really tightly) but I do believe Ciara admitted that she also enjoyed the evening. What each individual gained from that evening was wonderful to hear and see. The plans for the future as a Stoma group in Kerry, the ideas that Ciara has shared with the group and impact of her courage will always be appreciated.

Although it may not be the most ideal situation one thought they would find themselves in, Ciara is the proof that relationships can develop, and support is available for any patient with a stoma. You are never alone.

The Next Six Months

To be honest I knew the odds were stacked against me, but at the same time it was a bit of a blow to find that chemotherapy did not work for me. I was told that maybe I had a year to a year and a half.

I thank my very lucky stars that I was not alone on the day I received that news. I had my brother Shane with me who is an absolute rock!

I had only met my main oncologist three or four times, and I really felt that I needed some extra support, so I asked Mr Rice, if he had the time, to come with me for the appointment; I knew the news might be bad. To my surprise, he did and sat near me throughout the consultation. I was so grateful to him because the one thing I have learned in all this is support, both emotional and physical, is very important. It doesn't matter where you get it from, it doesn't have to be a doctor, but even the strongest of the strong will need someone for support coping with this disease.

I count myself very lucky to have had such great support in my life between my family, friends and medical team. I do not know what I did in this life time to deserve such a great doctor like Mr Rice. He has been more like a friend and the greatest support to me during the six months going in to see him. His positivity and his outlook on life got me out of the black fog that I was living in. He made me realise you live for now, not for the future, and to enjoy every second of life. I got my smile back, thanks to him.

A Note from Mr. John Rice

Orthopaedic Surgeon

In August 2012, I accompanied Ciara and her brother Shane to a consultation with Dr. Moylan, who in a very nice clinical fashion explained that chemotherapy obviously wasn't working in controlling the spread of the cancer within Ciara's lungs and therefore he felt further chemotherapy was not indicated.

It was my privilege to be with Ciara and Shane at the time of this devastating news however, Ciara's bravery was commendable at that time and I was impressed that her concern lay with the wellbeing of her family, and with other patients, both now and in the future who would be affected with Osteosarcoma.

Ciara was more concerned about others than with her own plight and this was a characteristic that is very rare and commendable.

Over the last few months, Ciara has not had any active treatment for her cancer. She attends the Orthopaedic Clinic on a monthly basis. We have serial x-rays of her chest and amazingly tumours in her past chest x rays haven't shown significant progression. Ciara remains in good form and I look forward to our monthly meetings at the Outpatients of Kerry General Hospital. We have a good chat and recognise the importance of living life and getting the most from one day at a time. The consultations with Ciara are good for me to appreciate the we live life for the present and it is a good idea not to look too far into the future.

Now

In many ways it is the end of the world being terminally ill. My life is being cut short. I am not going to see my nephews and nieces grow up, will miss out on the highlights of their lives. My mind keeps posing the big question, will they remember me?

And yet I have had a good life, have many very good friends and a brilliant family behind me. I can`t deny that I have had one or two dreams work out for me, just in case you are wondering!! During my Animal Care course in Cork I was lucky enough to spend some work experience segment of that course in Fota Wildlife Park. I made friends with all the giraffes and finally experienced some close proximity to cheetahs in the Park.

I have also been lucky enough to change careers and return to college, which resulted in me being employed in the Laboratory in Vistakon, where I have been fortunate enough to meet many more new good friends.

I also had the opportunity to go and see Andrea Bocelli live in the O2, which was brilliant. So I must be thankful, for I have in a sense lived more than one life.

The key, as I have come to understand, is to be thankful for what you have got and to never take life for granted. Naturally I am scared of the end and of what is to come, but I am determined to enjoy every minute and keep a big smile on my face and enjoy the days that are left to me with my family and friends. In a strange way I even look forward to my monthly consults with Mr Rice, though I am nervous of what the next x-ray will show.

The Colostomy has been a blessing in disguise as fortunately I have had no issues in being house bound or any confidence problems. I had a few typical issues like a hernia, which involved minor surgery to sort out. I have learned if you wear appropriate protective gear it helps to prevent any future hernias. I have had no other serious issues with living with a stoma. I also found that your stoma Nurse is your very vital best friend who is a mountain of information and great support.

July 2013

I have now just been told I have a few weeks to live, while yes it is a scary time, I find it is harder for my family and friends than for myself. I have the main man himself looking after me as well as the lovely Dr

156

Sheehan, what more could I ask for. The one thing I do find hard is trying to breath normally.

It is my hope that reading my story will increase awareness of this terrible disease that is Osteosarcoma. I hope that it will help someone to cope with this disease.

A good relationship built up, whether it is with your GP or your consultant, is important because you need to feel comfortable talking to your doctor about anything i.e. the most intimate problems like incontinence or bowel problems etc. Your doctor cares and is well used to talking about these matters and there is no shame in it. Before being diagnosed I would have been embarrassed to talk about these types of issues , but the relationship I have with my GP and my Consultant meant that I could talk to them about anything. All doctors are the same; it is what they are trained for. So please do not feel embarrassed or shy because these caring professionals will help you if ever you need them.

My faith remains strong in science, one day a cure will be found. I sign off urging people to get the bottom of any unexplained and persistent pain.

Sadly, Ciara lost her long battle with osteosarcoma on July 25th 2013. She passed peacefully surrounded by her family and friends.

Osteosarcoma Information -

Prof. Carney and Dr. Grainne O'Kane

Osteosarcoma is one of the most common primary malignant tumours of bone, occurring with an incidence of 2-3 per million per year, with an average of 10 cases per year in Ireland. It occurs more frequently in young adults and has a male to female ratio of 1.4.

The most commonly affected sites include the long bones around the knee joint (femur, tibia) and the humerus. Others such as spinal osteosarcoma tend to occur in older adults. Osteosarcoma of the jaw can occur but is rare. There are a number of different histological subtypes of osteosarcoma which are all characterised by cancer cells producing osteoid. Osteosarcoma can also be classified as localised (confined to affected bone only) or metastatic (spread to other sites). The most common site for metastases are the lungs.

In most cases the exact cause of osteosarcoma is unknown. Some rare genetic diseases such as Li Fraumeni syndrome can result in development of cancers including osteosarcoma. In older patients pre existing bone problems such as Paget's disease and fibrous dysplasia can increase your risk.

Patients often present with pain followed by swelling and limited joint movement. Very often these symptoms can be mistaken for simple bone pain or muscle strain. Plain x-rays can reveal changes in bone characteristic of osteosarcoma and is an important part of the initial work up. If presentation and investigations are suggestive of osteosarcoma, referral should be made to the appropriate centre as the correct diagnosis and multidisciplinary team management will aid in curing such patients.

Following referral, patients undergo a number of more definitive tests including an MRI scan of the affected bone/joint, bloods and usually a staging CT scan to assess the lungs. These tests are organised conjointly with the orthopaedic surgeon and oncologist. A biopsy of the tumour is a very important part of the diagnostic work up and should be done by the surgeon planning to operate on the patient.

The treatment of this uncommon tumour requires input from a number of specialists. Standard of care includes chemotherapy (oncology) followed by surgery (orthopaedics) followed by further chemotherapy. Surgeons will plan the operation very carefully. Most patients will have 'limb sparing' surgery which means the tumour and part of bone can be removed and a prosthesis inserted. Some patients however will require an amputation in order to fully remove all cancer cells and provide the best possible outcome for the patient in the long term. The type of surgery depends on a number of factors including the cancer site, proximity to blood vessels and how much the tumour has responded to chemotherapy.

Chemotherapy plays a very important role in the management of osteosarcoma and has increased the survival at 5 years from 20% with surgery alone to 70% with combined treatment. Chemotherapy given before surgery can help treat any secondary's that haven't been detected and can help the surgeon perform 'limb sparing' surgery. It also provides the oncologist with important information on the cancer cells. Cancers that show a lot of cell death at surgery can continue to be treated with the same chemotherapy after surgery. However those cancers that do not may require a change in the chemotherapy.

Predicting which patients will be cured from their disease can be difficult but a number of factors are known to contribute. Patients with metastases at the time of diagnosis tend to do poorly as do patients older than 40 years. Clearing all cancer at the time of surgery helps prevent recurrence at the same site. Importantly those patients whose tumours do not respond well to chemotherapy before surgery also have a worse outcome.

In patients with lung metastases cure is only possible if these can be resected. Such cases require discussion at a multidisciplinary team meeting.

In patients who have lots of secondary's or inoperable disease, treatment with chemotherapy is palliative and given in attempt to prolong life and improve quality of life. The investigations and treatment of osteosarcoma should be performed only at large centralised centres who have experience in this area.

Tributes to Ciara

Growing up with Ciara

Being an only sister to two older brothers, Ciara at times was seen as a 'foreigner' by us boys. Ciara was quick to learn she had to fight her corner, a trait that stands to her today, and fight we did, about what, I do not know! What does stand out for me is how we were made to make-up or were punished after a fight. I don't know how many lollipops or ice-creams were taken off me and given to Ciara (and vice versa), both being sent to bed early on a summers evening is particularly cruel.

One vivid punishment was my 1985 collection of Manchester United player posters, a season long exploit of match and shoot magazine to get the full team. I remember using my airplane model paint to start a career in street graffiti, thinking starting small scale like on a Dolls House was the way to go. An eye for an eye .... that was the last time Bryan Robson, Norman Whiteside and Jasper Olsen graced my wall.

It's funny then that Manchester United or more

accurately the career of Roy Keane is something Ciara and I would have followed together closely later in life, maybe it was the Cork blood or the never give up attitude of Roy that we both felt a kindred spirit. Many a long conversation filled the day with Roy this and Roy that, well before 'World War Saipan'. In further regard to footy as we grew older Ciara always became an option if we were 1 short for a kick around – last option kind of thing and as she got better to holding down a regular spot on our indoor soccer nights, a tight man-marker who you always knew got something on the ball or the man ...... bit like her idol !!

Having a 'fighting' daughter and son myself with a similar age gap, reminds me to remember the trials as fondly as the tribulations.

Ciara is definitely not spiritual – so she is not going to like this one. On a family trip to that 1980 craze – The moving statue I have a vivid memory.

An hour long car journey - A 3 mile walk after giving a farmer 5 pound to 'mind' the car - 3000 people on the side of a hill over-looking the Grotto – Giant loud speakers all over the hillside – the drone of the crowd responses 'Pray for Us'. No this was not Craggy Island it was Ballinspittle Cork 1986.

I stood up on the hill about a half a kilometre back and can remember Ciara kneeling directly in front of the statue with a pile of similarly aged kids. But the

164

extraordinary moment was on the way home out of the blue she piped up from the middle of the back seat (another thing we fought like cats and dogs over) that Holy Mary had spoken to her. Ciara had been having, to me as a 10 year old 'wet the bed problems' but I believe they were Kidney infections at the time. So Holy Mary told her she would never have trouble wetting the bed again ... and she didn't. Now while Ciara is vehemently denying this one, let me remind her, she took the confirmation name Maria as a result of this episode.

Aidan O'Neill.

Our friend

It was the Summer of '91 and my neighbour Fr. Padraig Kennelly had been ordained a priest. Little did I know that this event would lead to me meeting my best friend. Fr. Padraig said mass in my aunt Kathleens house and it was there that I met Ciara. Ciara had kindly offered to paint Kathleens gate, even aged ten Ciara had a heart of gold, and so Kathleen invited her to mass.

We were introduced and chatted happily all night. I remember that I was asked to sing. I was and still am totally tone deaf but being ten and foolish I decided to give it a go. I was a bag of nerves before my solo performance but my brand new friend coached me, dished out sound advice (a trend that would continue into adulthood), said she would say a poem too and that we'd both be great. Well I wasn't and halfway through my rendition of" the fields of Athenry" I was requested to stop! Ciara comforted me and that sealed the deal...a fantastic friendship was formed.

Despite being in different primary schools we spent every weekend and school holidays together. Our childhood was spent walking greyhounds, playing with barbies and collecting soaps. We were inseparable and despite mammoth arguments we got on like a house on fire! We once rescued a kitten from a stream and argued for a day over who would keep it. Ciara won and Sasha as she was christened lived to a ripe old age.

Our friendship continued into teenage years where we both attended Presentation Convent secondary school in Listowel. We had some fun!! We were both social butterflies and loved going out. We never missed a night in the Atlantic nightclub in Ballybunion during the Summer and Quilters bar in Listowel in Winter, so much so that Ciaras aunt Sheila, christened us "party ladies". Yes indeed us ladies sure enjoyed ourselves. Any mad, cracked notion that I had, Ciara usually thought it was a good idea and vice versa. It

166

was these cracked notions that led to us walking home from Ballybunion in strappy sandals or getting locked in a portaloo in Cork!

We went to college in separate counties, Ciara in Cork and me in Limerick but despite the long distance and new circles of friends Ciara was always my closest confidante- the person I turned to when I needed a shoulder to cry on or a good laugh. I got married in 2003 and Ciara was my maid of honour. It was my honour to have such a special friend at my side on that day.

Ciara was a truly wonderful friend- fiercely loyal, kind and caring but also pragmatic, dishing out sound advice when needed. Her loyalty was tremendous and once Ciara was your friend she was forever in your corner. Ciara had a kindness and generosity of spirit that knew no bounds.

Ciara is the bravest person I know and she dealt with her illness with such strength and dignity that at times it blew me away. She remained that positive, kind hearted person until the end. With Ciara's passing I lost one of my best friends and I feel that loss deeply. Ciara's friendship is a true blessing in my life and I am so privileged to be able to call her my friend . Friends like Ciara are a rare gift but it's a gift that I will always treasure.

Margaret Flahive

167

Ciara was my dear friend. She was one of the most courageous people I know. Some of the words that spring to mind are brave, strong, funny and stubborn. Her spirit and strength got her through the last three years with courage and grace.

Ciara was full of life. Even before her illness she really enjoyed life. During her illness she was determined to make the most of every minute, she was always up for a laugh. If I wasn't in good form she would be full of mischief, poking and prodding me and winding me up until she got a response.

She was strong willed and could be stubborn and dig her heels in. If she liked you, she liked you and there was no better friend to have .That strong will and fighting spirit is what got her through... and her sense of humour.

She loved animals. Her dogs were a big part of her life. She was there for them and they for her always.

Ciara liked to drive. We'd often go to Ballybunion for a spin and drop into the Feale Bar for a 'coffee' and a game of cards on the way home. Ciara didn't like to loose! We'd visit Kylemore strand where Ciara loved to take photos of sea birds in flight, waves and pebbles in the sand.

Countless cups of tea and coffee and lots of chat

were a big part of Ciara's, her mum's and my life over the past three years. Peggy would make the coffee and bring it down to us and we'd chat away. Those are the simple, precious memories that I will treasure about Ciara.

Rest in Peace Ciara
Le Grá, Niamh

Ciara and I first met many years ago when she came to the veterinary practice on work experience from her animal care course. Through our shared love of animals, we became firm friends. Ciara was passionate about all types of animals. Her greatest loves were for the big cats and of course her two beautiful German Shepherds, Strider and Chan. We spent many a happy hour down Ballyseedy woods with our combined pack of dogs.

Ciara's strength and courage is an inspiration to all who knew her. She was always more concerned about her family and friends, and how her illness affected us. She rarely complained, despite everything that she had to endure.

Throughout her own struggle she worked hard to increase awareness of osteosarcoma through her A Friend in Need Facebook page, which was an information and support page for all types of cancer. She leaves as her legacy, the story of her journey and as per her wishes, the proceeds of this book will be divided equally between Kerry General Hospital – who gave her such excellent care and Osteosarcoma research, with the hope that her contribution will help patients in the future. That was typical Ciara, always thinking about how she could help others, despite her own plight.

I count myself extremely lucky to have had Ciara in my life, she was a really decent person, and a really good friend. She will be sorely missed.

Karen Davison